Atlas of Non-Invasive Coronary Angiography by Multidetector Computed Tomography

Developments in Cardiovascular Medicine

Previous volumes are still available

Atlas of Non-Invasive Coronary Angiography by Multidetector Computed Tomography

edited by

Guillem Pons-Lladó, M.D.
Director, Cardiac Imaging Unit
Cardiology Department
Hospital de la Santa Creu I Sant Pau
Universitat Autónoma de Barcelona
Barcelona, Spain

Rubén Leta-Petracca, M.D.
Cardiac Imaging Unit
Cardiology Department
Hospital de la Santa Creu I Sant Pau
Universitat Autónoma de Barcelona
Barcelona, Spain

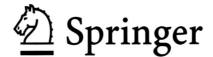 Springer

Guillem Pons-Lladó, M.D.
Director, Cardiac Imaging Unit
Cardiology Department
Hospital de la Santa Creu I Sant Pau
Universitat Autónoma de Barcelona
Barcelona, Spain

Rubén Leta-Petracca, M.D.
Cardiac Imaging Unit
Cardiology Department
Hospital de la Santa Creu I Sant Pau
Universitat Autónoma de Barcelona
Barcelona, Spain

Library of Congress Control Number: 2006922022

ISBN-13: 978-0-387-33044-0
ISBN-10: 0-387-33044-5

e-ISBN-13: 978-0-387-33048-8
e-ISBN-10: 0-387-33048-8

Printed on acid-free paper.

9 8 7 6 5 4 3 2 1

springer.com

Chapter 5: *Morphological and Functional Assessment of Heart Chambers by MDCT* 113

Guillem Pons-Lladó

Index

List of Contributors

Xavier Alomar-Serrallach, M.D. Radiology Department, Clínica Creu Blanca, Barcelona, Spain

Ernesto Castillo-Gallo, M.D. CT & MR Department, Instituto Radiológico Castillo, Madrid, Spain

Francesc Carreras-Costa, M.D. Cardiac Imaging Unit, Cardiology Department, Hospital de la Santa Creu i Sant Pau, Clínica Creu Blanca, Barcelona, Spain

Rubén Leta-Petracca, M.D. Cardiac Imaging Unit, Cardiology Department, Hospital de la Santa Creu i Sant Pau, Clínica Creu Blanca, Barcelona, Spain

Guillem Pons-Lladó, M.D. Cardiac Imaging Unit, Cardiology Department, Hospital de la Santa Creu i Sant Pau, Clínica Creu Blanca, Barcelona, Spain

Sandra Pujadas-Olano, M.D. Cardiac Imaging Unit, Cardiology Department, Hospital de la Santa Creu i Sant Pau, Clínica Creu Blanca, Barcelona, Spain

The field of noninvasive imaging of cardio-vascular disorders has advanced considerably in recent years, particularly with the introduction of Cardiovascular Magnetic Resonance (CMR), which has added its powerful resources to those of the extensively used echocardiographic techniques. While an actual integration of these two methods is still an ongoing issue in most clinical units, a new technique also appears on the horizon with promising perspectives: Multidetector Computed Tomography (MDCT), which has raised high expectations from its very first appearance, only a few years ago. Reasons for such an interest have been the superb resolution of images, providing a highly defined anatomical detail, and, as a consequence, the obtention of truly readable images of the coronary arteries.

Having a noninvasive coronary angiography available has been a much awaited goal for clinical cardiologists for decades. Ultrasound was earlier discarded for this purpose, while CMR has proven to be reliable in providing this information only in the most experienced hands and with methods of analysis submitted to continuous refinements. Thus, MDCT has found its place immediately after its arrival, filling a gap–imaging of the coronary arteries—which had been incompletely covered by former noninvasive techniques.

With such a well-provided panel of tools, diagnostic cardiology seems to have attained a point of excellence in the noninvasive assessment of patients with ischemic heart disease. On one side, echocardiography constitutes an essential tool for a routine scanning of patients with ischemic one or any other form of heart disease. CMR, on its part, contributes by means of accurately precise information, which is also unique in respect to the detection and quantitation of myocardial necrosis. Finally, MDCT has proven to be useful in providing detailed morphological information on coronary arteries. Although attractive, this scenario should not be considered, however, as inalterable. The very evolving nature of these techniques makes it difficult to anticipate with certainty which improvements will be introduced in the future and, what the prospects will be, even at midterm, in this field.

With a practical perspective, however, today MDCT coronary angiography constitutes an indispensable tool that should be mastered by every department active on cardiac imaging. The aim of this Atlas is to provide with an extensive body of images taken with a Toshiba Aquilion system (most of them from a 64-slice unit) an illustration of the capacities of the technique for the analysis of the anatomy of coronary arteries. A detailed text accompanying the figures and an updated list of references will guide the reader throughout his/her initiation to the technique.

An effective management strategy of the different resources available for cardiac imaging implies new changing attitudes with respect to those deeply rooted in some medical specialties, as cardiology or radiology. Cardiac MDCT is a good example of a technique with an extremely useful potential that, in order to be adequately exploited, requires an unreserved cooperation between professionals from both sides. Cardiologists and radiologists have both cooperated in writing this Atlas, as they usually do in everyday practice with cardiac MDCT, each of them contributing with complementary roles. Receiving the patient, setting the system, performing the exam, reconstructing volumes, and a first reporting of the studies are tasks under the radiological domain, in addition to the important issue of an authorized reading of images to rule out abnormal noncardiac findings in the thoracic volume acquired. A definitive reporting and, particularly, the integration of findings of the exam on the whole clinical process of the patient, are responsibilities of the cardiological team, together with the important issue of defining and selecting the indications for the studies. With this perspective, we do firmly believe that the constitution of integrated Cardiac Imaging units will be a widespread practice in the near future as the optimal approach to deal with all aspects of this increasingly demanding field, and for the benefit of patients with cardiovascular disease.

Guillem Pons-Lladó, M.D.
Cardiac Imaging Unit
Cardiology Department
Hospital de la Santa Creu i Sant Pau
Clínica Creu Blanca
Barcelona, Spain

Basics and Performance of Cardiac Computed Tomography

1

XAVIER ALOMAR-SERRALLACH
ERNESTO CASTILLO-GALLO
GUILLEM PONS-LLADÓ

1.1 Introduction

The recent introduction of Multidetector Computed Tomography (MDCT) represents a milestone in the evolution of Computed Tomography, that started in the decade of 1970. Faster velocities of acquisition, higher spatial and temporal resolution, and better image quality are advantages of MDCT over the former single-slice systems that allow the development of cardiac applications on a realistic basis. MDCT also implies a different way of analysis of the information by the radiologist; the availability of a true anatomical volume through which the operator may navigate and easily reconstruct planar images has been made possible by the technological advance of computers. This derives in a potentially high complexity of studies, particularly those of the heart, that requires an adequate level of expertise from the specialist in charge. For this reason, a truly efficient outcome of these studies can only be attained when there is a close cooperation between cardiologists and radiologists. While cardiologists may provide a useful clinical perspective and competent image analysis, an in-depth knowledge of the potential and technical resources of MDCT can only be gained from a radiological view. The concepts developed in this chapter are aimed to cover this aspect.

1.2 Historical Perspective of Computed Tomography

Basic to the MDCT technology are the theoretical principles of reconstruction of a three-dimensional (3D) object from multiple two-dimensional (2D) views relying on a complex mathematical model, as formulated by Johann Radon in 1917. The lack of computer facilites prevented this theory from being brought into practice at that time. The first system of CT was devised in 1972[1] after the work of Allan Cormack and Godfrey Hounsfield, for which they were laureated with the Noble Prize in Physiology and Medicine in 1979.[2]

Early systems were provided with an X-ray tube and a two–slice detector built opposite each other into a rotating device, performing acquisitions at every degree of rotation up to 180°, which constituted the full span of rotation, after which an axial slice was reconstructed. The image thus obtained had a matrix of 80 × 80 pixels, with the acquisition time (temporal resolution) being over 5 minutes. In despite of these rather modest features, CT images proved to be able to distinguish between tissue components of organic structures with slighly different attenuation to X-ray.

Continuous technical improvements allowed a reduction of the temporal resolution to less than 5 seconds, and the sequential acquisition of a series of parallel axial slices when combining the acquisition with measured displacements of the table. The addition of an electrocardiographic synchronization led to the obtention of still images of the heart[3] in the early 1980's.

An outstanding innovation for the study of the heart was introduced in 1982[4] with the electron-beam CT (EBCT). This system does not present with an X-ray emission source or any rotational element into the gantry, but with a focused electron beam in stationary tungsten targets, thus permitting very rapid scanning times. A dramatic reduction of temporal resolution to 50–100 msec. for an axial slice, and a slice thickness at the submillimetric level (0.8 mm) made possible the obtention of images useful for the detection and quantification of calcium in the coronary arterial wall[5], and with the aid of an X-ray opaque contrast agent, for the obtention of the first noninvasive coronary angiography studies[6]. A major drawback of EBCT has been the high cost of both the purchase of the system and its maintenance, which has greatly limited widespread use of this technique.

The introduction of CT technology based on the so-called spiral or helical acquisition, late in the 1980's, also represented an important step. In these systems, a sliding ring containing both the X-ray emitting source and the detectors allows a fast continuous rotation of the gantry that sweeps the body of the patient in a helical course as the table is continually moving in the direction of the longitudinal axis[7]. The rotation time of the gantry was initially of 1 sec., while in 1994 it had been reduced to 0.75 sec., this allowing for the first time a true volumetric acquisition of an anatomical region in 25–30 sec. with slices between 2–10 mm thick[7]. Despite these features, however, the obtention of adequate images of the heart and the coronary arteries was still beyond the scope of CT.

An important advance was the introduction, in 1993, of multidetector computer tomography (MDCT) technology. Systems initially had 2 rows of detectors[9], this reducing the time of the examination, which was only appropriate for the study of the heart. Then, systems equipped with 4 rows of parallel detectors were available, in 1998, providing rotation times of 0.5 sec. and, by means of complex segmentation algorithms, reconstructions with a temporal resolution between 125–250 msec.[10] Spatial resolution was also improved as slice thickness was reduced to 1–1.25 mm. With these advances, the obtention of a cardiac volume free of movement artifacts was possible, although this implied a breath-hold time between 35–45 sec.

Systems with 8, 12 and 16 rows of detectors soon followed, the latter becoming available in 2002, for the first time allowing, the obtention of cardiac volume with a true isotropic spatial resolution: identical size of the voxel in the three planes, between 0.5–0.625 mm, and with rotation time below 0.5 sec.[11-13] Temporal resolution for reconstructed volumes has been reduced to 53–65 msec., which is within the range of values rendered by EBCT systems. The required breath-hold time for 16-slice equipments is between 20–30 sec. Relevant as they are, these advancements have not been considered sufficient for cardiac examination, and during 2004–2005, new generations of MDCT equipped with 32, 40, and 64 detectors have been introduced[14]. The main advantage, in practice, of these new systems is the reduction in the scan time, allowing breath-hold times lower than 10 sec., which results in a high image quality for most studies that are otherwise free from arrhythmia or respiratory artifacts.

Future improvements will probably be made available with systems equipped with up to 256 detectors and, by means of flat panel digital detectors, allowing a reduction in spatial resolution to 0.2 mm, as has already been proven in animal studies[15].

1.3 Basic Principles of Multidetector Computed Tomography in the Study of the Heart

There are two main determinant aspects in the image quality of MDCT: spatial and temporal resolution, which, in turn, are dependent on the number of slices of the system, the extension of collimation, the rotation time, and the

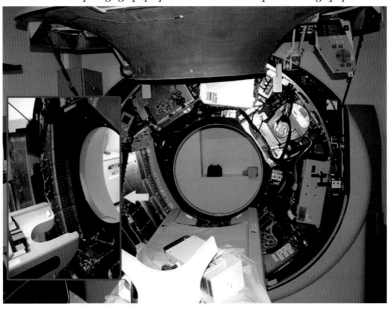

FIGURE 1.1 Vision of the components of an MDCT system: the inset shows a detail of the panel of detectors.

relationship between rotation time and table advancement (pitch). All of these are related with elements contained in the gantry of the system: the X-ray tube, and the detectors with collimators (Figure 1.1).

The scanning process consists of a constant movement of the table while the gantry rotates and continuously emits X-rays. There is an attenuation of rays by tissues depending on their density, which is received by the detectors, the final image consisting on an attenuation map where every pixel has a value dependent on the tissue component. In despite of this apparent simplicity, the whole process is very complex in the case of MDCT. In those systems equipped with 16 rows, for instance, the number of detection elements or channels is between 14,000–16,000, and up to nearly 36,000 for some systems. These elements must be precisely read and digitized 1,000–2,000 times per second, the data then being processed and stored almost on real time by means of algorithms of interpolation and reconstruction techniques that demand fairly sophisticated computer equipment.

1.3.1 Detectors

The geometry of detectors is one of the aspects that has changed most significantly with the development of the different MDCT systems. The design of detectors is essential for an adequate slice thickness of the images. There are two modalities in the design of detectors:

fixed and adaptive-array (Figure 1.2). In the fixed-array design, the elements are identical in size, while in the adaptive-array those detectors situated in the centre of the field are smaller in size than those at the outer side. This allows an optimization between the acquisition time, slice thickness, and cone beam width. This, in turn, prevents the occurrence of artifacts in the peripheral region of the scan field in those studies requiring high spatial resolution, and, on the other hand, permits a reduction in the acquisition time in studies with standard spatial resolution.

1.3.2 Image reconstruction

There are two techniques of image reconstruction: ECG-triggered, or prospective scanning, and ECG-gated, or retrospective scanning.

In the prospective mode,[16] the scanning is performed at a predetermined time window on the cardiac cycle, usually during diastole (Figure 1.3). This time window can be defined in terms of milliseconds from the R wave of the ECG, or as a percentage of the cardiac cycle. It does not require a helical mode of acquisition, but every scan is performed after discrete displacements of the table. The minimum data for the image formation is obtained in a fraction of the complete rotation of the gantry (usually 240°–260°), by means of spatial interpolation algorithms. The effective temporal resolution of this mode is one half of the rotation time of the

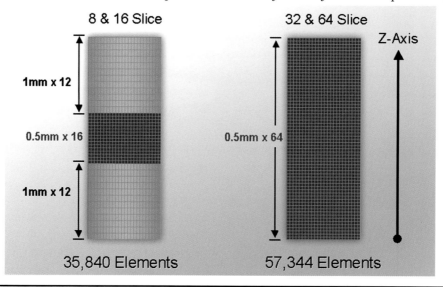

FIGURE 1.2 Diagrams depicting the arrangement of detectors in adaptive (left) and fixed (right) modes of array (see text for explanation). *Courtesy of Toshiba Medical Systems.*

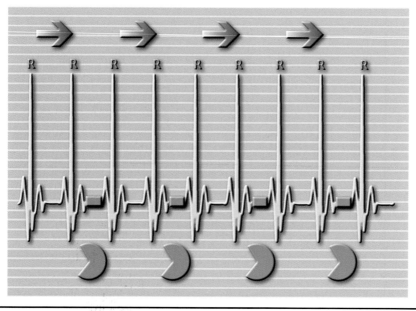

FIGURE 1.3 Prospective scanning method, showing the window of acquisition during diastole. *Courtesy of Toshiba Medical Systems.*

system (half-scan reconstruction), thus allowing a reduction in the acquisition time and in the radiation dose. However, there is a limitation on the minimal slice thickness with this mode—to 2.5–3 mm—in order to maintain a reasonable breath-hold time. In practice, the prospective mode of reconstruction is applied in the study of coronary artery calcium.

In retrospective scanning,[17] the acquisition is performed in a continuous helical mode during one breath-hold. A simultaneous recording of the ECG allows for a posterior reconstruction of images at determined phases of the whole cardiac cycle, but from different cycles-segmented reconstruction (Figure 1.4). Heart rate is a crucial aspect in this mode, as the more cardiac cycles that are present in the breath-hold period, the higher the number of segments available for the image reconstruction, thus improving the temporal resolution. A changing

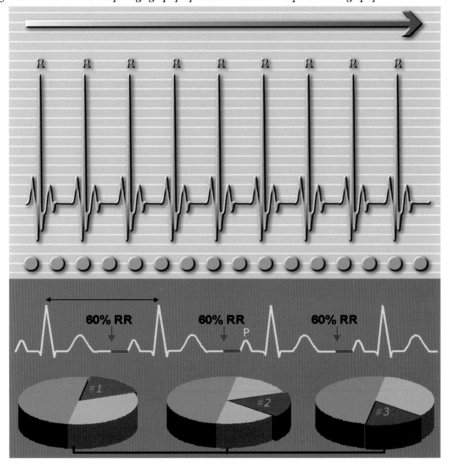

FIGURE 1.4 Retrospective scanning method: diagrams of the continuous helical acquisition (upper panel) and the segmented reconstruction (lower panel). *Courtesy of Toshiba Medical Systems.*

heart rate during the short period of scan may be a potential technical limitation for this mode of acquisition. Continuous acquisition in the restrospective scanning leads to a higher radiation dose than in the prospective mode. However, spatial resolution is optimal in this modality, as slice thickness may be reduced to 0.5 mm. Retrospective scanning is thus the adequate mode of acquisition for coronary angiography, as well as for the study of left ventricular function, provided the acquisition of data over the whole cardiac cycle is continuous.

1.3.3 Temporal resolution

The time interval where every acqustion of data is performed is referred to as temporal resolution. This is a crucial point in cardiac imaging, due to the constant movement of the heart itself. In CT, temporal resolution is directly related to the rotation time of the gantry and the segmented reconstruction software available. In modern MDCT equipment, rotation time is between 330–400 msec., which is too long a time length to obtain an axial plane of the heart devoid of moving artifacts. Different strategies have been devised to deal with this limitation. Reconstruction using data acquired in one-half of the rotation time (half-scan) reduces temporal resolution to 165–200 msec., which is still too long for cardiac imaging, as the maximal length of time for obtaining a motionless image of the heart is nearly 50 msec.[18] Segmental reconstruction, on the other hand, has represented a substantial improvement, as temporal resolution can be further reduced to such value.[19]

1.3.4 Spatial resolution

Defined as the ability to distinguish between two adjacent points in terms of distance, in the case of a volumetric technique such as MDCT, this concept must be referred to in both the axial direction (in-plane, XY) and the longitudinal direction (Z axis). In practice, spatial resolution in the axial direction is expressed as the size of the pixel in the image. Standard values in cardiac MDCT, provided by an image matrix of 512×512 elements and a field-of-view of 200–250 mm, give an in-plane resolution of 0.35–0.45 mm, which is nearly equal to the resolution attained in the longitudinal Z axis, this being determined by the width of detectors.

The element of the image is then called a voxel which, in this case, is isotropic in size (Figure 1.5).

1.3.5 Control of radiation dose

The amount of radiation absorbed by the patient during a MDCT study of the heart is considerable. The biological effect and risk estimation of the ionizing radiation received is expressed as "effective dose" in miliSievert (mSv). Table 1.1 presents documented values of

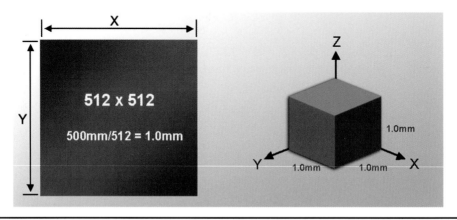

FIGURE 1.5 Isotropic voxel: a field-of-view of 500 mm and an image matrix of 512×512 results in a squared pixel size of 1 mm on the $x–y$ axis (left panel); a slice thickness of 1 mm gives a final isotropic voxel on the $x–y–z$ dimension (right panel). *Courtesy of Toshiba Medical Systems.*

Table 1.1 Values of mean effective radiation doses in natural and diagnostic exposures[20–22]. EBCT: electron beam computed tomography; MIBI: methoxyisobutyl isonitrile; SPECT: single photon emission computed tomography; Tc: technetium; Tl: thallium.

Exposure	Effective dose (mSv)	
Natural environmental radiation	2–5/year	
Transoceanic flight	0.1 (per flight)	
Chest X-ray (2 projections)	0.04–0.06	
Coronary angiography (diagnostic)	2–10	
Coronary angiography (interventional)	25	
Myocardial SPECT (^{99m}Tc –MIBI)	10	
Myocardial SPECT (^{201}Tl)	23	
Cranial CT	1–2	
Thoracic CT (4-slice)	12–13	
Abdominal CT (4-slice)	15–16	
	Calcium score	Coronary angiography
Cardiac EBCT	0.8–1.3	1.5–2
Cardiac MDCT (4-slice)	1.5–6.2	3–13
Cardiac MDCT (8-slice)	2.9–3.6	11.8–24.2
Cardiac MDCT (32-64-slice)	2.9–3.6	9–24

effective doses for MDCT and other common diagnostic procedures.[20–22] The effective dose resulting from a MDCT exam is variable, depending on several factors such as the size of the acquired volume, pitch (as an indirect measure of the exposure time), and intensity (expressed in mAs) of the X-ray emission. The issue of radiation has lead manufacturers to introduce methods for reducing the doses emitted by the equipment. These include tube modulation systems, aimed at reducing the X-ray emission in nontarget areas or during particular phases of the cardiac cycle.

There is no safety range in terms of radiation dose for the development of cancer. Population studies[23] have suggested that there is a risk with current diagnostic X-ray tests, although rates of malignancy attributable to these tests are within an acceptable range, provided the advantages of its rational use.

1.4 Performance of a Cardiac MDCT Study

1.4.1 Preparation of the patient

Essential to the obtention of an adequate study is the ability of the patient to perform a breath-hold and the maintenance of a stable heart rate. Reassurance of the patient from the entrance to the scanning room must be a rule, including an appropriate knowledge of the whole process. Mild oral sedation with sublingual diazepam (5 mg) can be added in particularly anxious individuals.

As with every study involving the administration of contrast, a history of hypersensitivity to iodinated contrast media must be ruled out. Previous acute or chronic renal failure has to be considered and managed by forms of renal protection protocols, including adequate fluid intake, administration of n-acetylcysteine, or the use of contrast agents with a potentially reduced nephrotoxic effect[24]. In cases with a formal contraindication to iodinated agents, gadolinium compounds have been used as an alternative[25].

A stable venous line must be available, this requiring a 18-to-20 gauge needle placed into an antecubital vein. Finally, the preparation for the study must include a pre-exam testing of the ability of the patient for sustaining a breath-hold long enough for the purposes of the examination. In addition, this allows a checking of potential heart rate variability during the breath-hold period. In cases with wide heart rate variation or with frequent premature contractions during apnea, the administration of oxygen through nasal cannulae during the acquisition can reduce these events, thus improving image quality. The administration of beta-blocking agents (metoprolol) has been recommended in patients with relatively fast heart rates (65–70 b.p.m.) for increasing the diastolic phase of the cardiac cycle, which facilitates the acquisition process. At present, however, the improvement in the segmented reconstruction algorithms allows a ready acquisition even at high heart rates, without a premedication with these agents.

1.4.2 Image acquisition and contrast administration

A first step in the imaging process is to delineate the limits of the acquisition. This is accomplished by the obtention of the so-called scanogram (Figure 1.6). Based on the anatomical information from this scan, a second acquisition, also without contrast administration, is planned encompassing the region between the tracheal carina and the upper third of the liver. This ECG-triggered prospective scan is aimed to assess the presence and extent of calcium in the coronary artery walls (Figure 1.7). Analysis and quantitation of coronary artery calcium is discussed in Chapter 3.

The acquisition for the coronary angiography is also prescribed on the scanogram, where the region of interest can be delineated. As an angiographic study, it requires the administration of a contrast agent to enhance the vascular tree. The volume of contrast depends on the acquisition time of the equipment. For those systems with 64 detectors, the total volume given is 65–75 cc. In all cases, the administration of the contrast should be fast (4–5 cc/s) in order to more reliably enhance the vascular bed. Important in this sense is the obtention of images during the arterial phase of the contrast injection.

For this purpose, the start of the acquisition must be triggered with the arrival of contrast to the aortic root by means of a bolus tracking technique (Figure 1.8). This consists of a continuous scan on a single axial slice. On this image, a region of interest is placed at the aortic level which examines the Hounsfield units during the passage of the contrast agent. When a predeterminate value of units is accomplished (130–150 HU), this indicating an appropriate

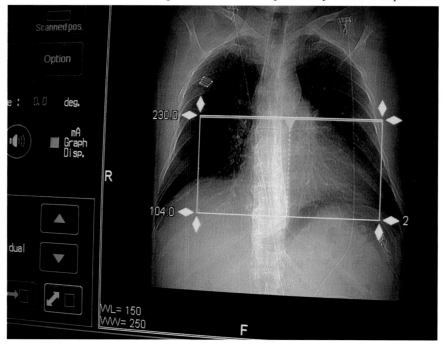

FIGURE 1.6 Scanogram delineating the limits of the acquisition volume.

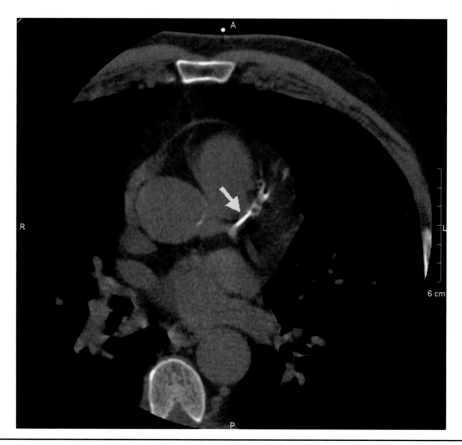

FIGURE 1.7 Noncontrast prospective scan showing a coronary arterial wall calcification (arrow) at the level of the left anterior descending artery.

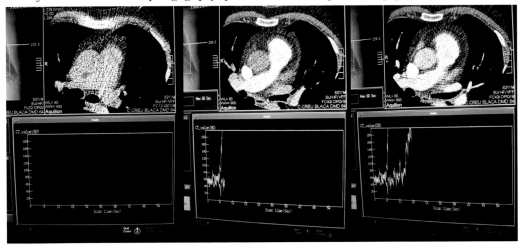

FIGURE 1.8 Bolus tracking technique: regions of interest (ROIs) are positioned on the pulmonary artery and on the ascending aorta that indicate the precise moment of arrival of the contrast agent. Upper panels show an axial slice showing the temporal changes in density at the great vessels. Lower panels show the plot of density (y axis, in Hounsfield units) of both ROIs over time (x axis, in seconds).

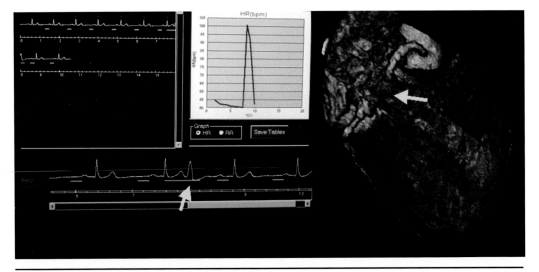

FIGURE 1.9 The presence of a premature beat during the acquisition (arrow on the left panel), detected as a sudden increase in heart rate, induces an artifact in the 3D volume rendering image (arrow on the right panel).

opacification of the aortic root, the acquisition of the whole cardiac volume is started. The total duration of the acquisition, and thus of the breath-hold period, is between 8–10 s in 64-slice systems to 25–30 s in 16-slice MDCT. Once this process is completed, the exam is finished and the patient can leave.

1.4.3 Image reconstruction

The reconstruction of images at the workstation is a time-consuming process, aimed to select the most appropriate set of images for coronary artery visualization[26], avoiding those reconstructions with artifacts due to cardiac motion. As a general rule, the phase of the cardiac cycle when the right coronary artery is best visualized is around 40% of the R-R period, while for the left coronary artery it is nearly 80%. A search centered on these intervals should then be started from the retrospective reconstruction of the whole cardiac cycle rendered by the system. The ECG recorded during the acquisition must be examined at this point to look for exaggerated cycle variability and/or premature beats that could introduce artifacts in the images (Figure 1.9). Current systems include facilities for arrhythmia rejection as automatic filters or manual editions of these premature beats. Important to note is that the exclusion of a premature beat from the reconstruction reduces the resolution of the images although the analysis may be feasible. The interpretation of the images, which is the final step of the process, is discussed in Chapter 4.

The information from the retrospective reconstruction of the whole cardiac cycle that is not considered for the study of the coronary vessels is not useless. Accordingly, the set of images that contain whole heart reconstructions gated at intervals between 5–10% of the cycle allows a cine format presentation constituted by 10–15 phases of the cardiac cycle. From this, a comprehensive exam of global and regional ventricular wall motion can be performed, as discussed in Chapter 5.

References

1. Hounsfield, G.N. Computerized transverse axial scanning (tomography).1. Description of system. *Br J Radiol*, 1973, 46, 1016–22.

2. Hounsfiled, G.N. Nobel award address: computed medical imaging. *Med Phys*, 1980, 7, 283–90.

3. Lackner, K., and P. Thurn. Computed Tomography of the heart: ECG-gated and continuous scans. *Radiology*, 1981, 140, 413–20.

4. Boyd, D.P., and M.J. Lipton. Cardiac computed-tomography. *Proc IEEE*, 1983, 71, 298–307.

5. Agatston, A.S., et al. Quantification of coronary artery calcium using ultrafast computed tomography. *J Am Coll Cardiol*, 1990, 15, 827–32.

6. Achenbach, S., W. Moshage, and K. Bachmann. Noninvasive coronary angiography by contrast-enhanced electron bean computed tomography. *Clin Cardiol*, 1998, 21, 323–30.

7. Kalender, W.A., et al. Spiral volumetric CT with single-breath-hold technique, continuous transport and continuous scanner rotation. *Radiology*, 1990, 176, 181–3.

8. Kalender, W.A. Thin-section three-dimensional spiral CT: is isotropic imaging possible? *Radiology*, 1995, 197, 578–80.

9. Liang, Y., and R.A. Kruger. Dual-slice spiral versus single-slice spiral scanning: comparison of the physical performance of two computed tomography scanners. *Med Phys*, 1996, 23, 205–20.

10. Nieman, K., et al. Coronary angiography with multi-slice computed tomography. *Lancet*, 2001, 357, 599–603.

11. Nieman, K., et al. Reliable noninvasive coronary angiography with fast submillimeter multislice spiral computed tomography. *Circulation*, 2002, 106, 2051–4.

12. Ropers, D., et al. Detection of coronary artery stenoses with thin-slice multi-detector row spiral computed tomography and multiplanar reconstruction. *Circulation*, 2003, 107, 664–6.

13. Leta, R., et al. Coronariografía no invasiva mediante tomografía computarizada con 16 detectores: estudio comparativo con la angiografía coronaria invasiva. *Rev Esp Cardiol*, 2004, 57, 217–24.

14. Nikolaou, K., et al. Advances in cardiac CT imaging: 64-slice scanner. *Int J Cardiovasc Imaging*, 2004, 20, 535–40.

15. Knollmann, F., and A. Pfoh. Image in cardiovascular medicine. Coronary artery imaging with flat-panel computed tomography. *Circulation*, 2003, 107, 1209.

16. Kachelriess, M., S. Ulzheimer, and W. Kalender. ECG-correlated image reconstruction from sub-second multi-slice spiral CT scans of the heart. *Med Phys*, 2000, 27, 1881–1902.

17. Woodhouse, C.E., W.R. Janowitz, and M. Viamonte Jr. Coronary arteries: retrospective cardiac gating technique to reduce cardiac motion artifact at spiral CT. *Radiology*, 1997, 204, 566–69.

18. Stehling, M.K., R. Turner, and P. Mansfield. Echo-planar imaging: magnetic resonance imaging in a fraction of a second. *Science*, 1991, 254, 43–50.

19. Flohr, T., and B. Ohnesorge. Heart rate adaptive optimization of spatial and temporal resolution for electrocardiogram-gated multislice spiral CT of the heart. *J Comput Assist Tomogr*, 2001, 25, 907–23.

20. Morin, R.L., T.C. Gerber, and C.H. McCollough. Radiation dose in computed tomography of the heart. *Circulation*, 2003, 107, 917–22.

21. Hunold, P., et al. Radiation exposure during cardiac CT: effective doses at multi-detector row CT and electron-beam CT. *Radiology*, 2003, 226, 145–52.

22. Jakobs, T.F., et al. Multislice helical CT of the heart with retrospective ECG gating: reduc-

tion of radiation exposure by ECG-controlled tube current modulation. *Eur Radiol*, 2002, 12, 1081–6.

23. Berrington de Gonzalez, A., and S. Darby. Risk of cancer from diagnostic X-rays: estimates for the UK and 14 other countries. *Lancet*, 2004, 363, 345–51.

24. Aspelin, P., et al. Nephrotoxicity in high-risk patients study of iso-osmolar and low-osmolar non-ionic contrast media study investigators. Nephrotoxic effects in high-risk patients under-

going angiography. *N Engl J Med*, 2003, 348, 491–9.

25. Strunk, H.M., and H. Schild. Actual clinical use of gadolinium-chelates for non-MRI applications. *Eur Radiol*, 2004, 14, 1055–62.

26. Lawler, L.P., H.K. Pannu, and E.K. Fishman. MDCT evaluation of the coronary arteries, 2004: how we do it—data acquisition, post-processing, display, and interpretation. *AJR Am J Roentgenol*, 2005, 184, 1402–12.

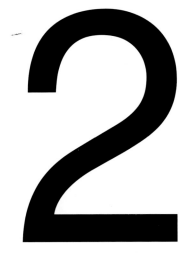

RUBÉN LETA-PETRACCA

Normal Anatomy and Congenital Abnormalities of the Coronary Arteries

2.1 Introduction

An adequate knowledge of the anatomy of coronary arteries and its normal variants is an important point for the analysis of MDCT images. Nomenclature of coronary anatomy is frequently confusing, as a number of anatomical, clinical and radiological terms are used in combination. This conventional terminology is useful, however, as it has been applied in conventional coronary angiography[1], and it will be maintained in the present chapter.

The heart is a highly differentiate blood vessel, with developed muscular walls. The vascular nutrition of myocardium is complex, with a number of anatomical normal variants that can involve even extracardiac vessels, such as bronchial, mammary and mediastinal arteries[2,3].

The coronary arteries are conductive vessels running through the epicardial surface of the heart, embedded in adipose tissue, and showing short segments of mild penetration into the myocardial tissue[3].

As indicated by its name (from the latin *corona*: wreath), coronary arteries are distributed over the heart as a crown-shape network, showing anastomotic communications between its different branches, particularly at the level of the base and the apex of the left ventricle. The connection between divisions of the same artery is known as homocollateral circulation, and the connection between different arteries is named heterocollateral circulation. Physiological collateral circulation acquires a relevant role in pathological circumstances[2].

Macroscopical appearance of coronary arteries is variable in terms of diameter, which is larger in the left artery than in the right one in more than half of individuals, while the opposite occurs in nearly 20%[2]. Also, the number of ramifications, its course—linear or sinusoid—(Figure 2.1), and the distance from the epicardial surface (Figure 2.2) is variable between individuals[3].

Coronary arteries emerge from the aorta through the coronary *ostia*, located at the right (or anterior) and the left (or left posterior) sinuses of Valsalva[2]. The coronary *ostia* (Figure 2.3) are situated at the level of the sinotubular junction or slightly below it (56% of cases), followed by a high left orifice and a low right orifice or at the level of the junction (30% of individuals)[4].

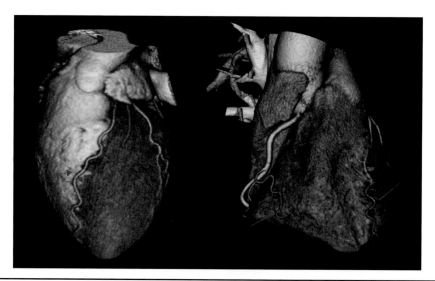

FIGURE 2.1

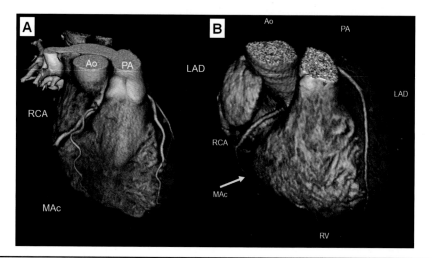

FIGURE 2.2

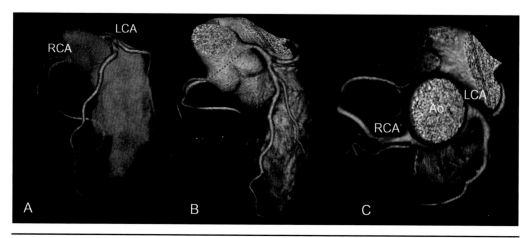

FIGURE 2.3

F. 2.1. Coronary arteries of tortuous course (arrows): this normal variant is frequently found in hypertensive patients.

F. 2.2. Differing distance of coronary arteries from epicardium: in patient A, the marginal acute (MAc) branch of the right coronary artery (RCA) courses close to the epicardium, while in patient B it runs at a distance from the external surface of the heart (arrow), this space being occupied by fat (deleted by filtering of the image). Ao: aorta; LAD: left anterior descending; PA: pulmonary artery; RV: right ventricle.

F. 2.3. Origin of the coronary arteries as seen from frontal (A and B) and cranial (C) views: observe that the right coronary *ostium* is anterior and caudal with respect to the left one, while both are equidistant from the coaptation point of the aortic valve (B panel). Ao: aorta; LCA: left coronary artery; RCA: right coronary artery.

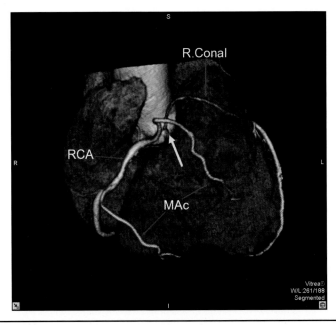

FIGURE 2.4 Independent origin of the right conal artery (yellow arrow). MAc: marginal acute; RCA: right coronary artery.

Although usually two coronary arteries (right and left) are seen emerging from the aorta, three or even four independent origins have been described. In these cases, frequently (36% of individuals) the right conal artery is the one with an independent origin[2] (Figure 2.4). Also, it is not rare to find separate origins for both main branches of the left artery, this implying the absence of left main trunk[4]. On the other hand, the origin of both arteries from a single coronary sinus has been described, either from a single *ostium* or from separate orifices at the same sinus[2].

2.2 Left Coronary Artery

The left coronary artery is a large artery (Figure 2.5) with an approximate diameter of 5 mm at its origin, that supplies an extensive portion of the walls of the left chambers of the heart, with blood including most of the interventricular septal mass[2].

2.2.1 Left main (LM) artery

A common initial segment of the left coronary artery, the LM has variable length (Figure 2.6), is embedded in adipose tissue, and courses between the main pulmonary artery and the left atrial appendage[3,5] (Figures 2.7–2.8). Rarely (<1% of individuals), the LM is absent (Figure 2.9), with independent origins of its main branches from the left coronary sinus[4].

In addition to its main ramification, the LM emits no other branches, except in those rare instances where the artery of the sinus node originates from it[2]. At the level of the left atrioventricular groove, the LM gives two or three

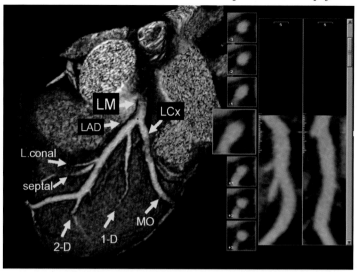

FIGURE 2.5 Left coronary artery with its branches, as seen on a 3D (left) and a multiplanar reconstruction (MPR) of its proximal segment (right). LAD: left anterior descending; L.Conal: left conal branch; LCx: left circumflex; LM: left main; MO: marginal obtuse branch of the LCx; Septal: first septal anterior branch of the LAD; 1D and 2D: first and second diagonal branches of the LAD.

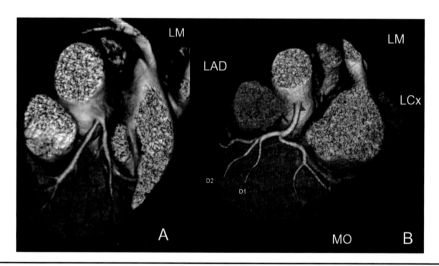

FIGURE 2.6 Short (A) and long (B) normal variants of left main (LM) coronary artery. LAD: left anterior descending; LCx: left circumflex; MO: marginal obtuse branch of the LCx; 1D and 2D: first and second diagonal branches of the LAD.

branches, namely the left anterior descending, the left circumflex artery and, occasionally, the intermediate artery[3].

2.2.2 Left anterior descending (LAD)

LAD coronary artery is a large vessel—4–5 mm in diameter at its proximal portion—that occupies the anterior interventricular groove, running in parallel with the great cardiac vein

(Figure 2.10), with which it exhibits crossover points[2,6]. It usually extends to the apical region of the left ventricle and, in two thirds of individuals, it reaches the distal (Figure 2.11) or even the middle portion of the posterior interventricular groove[7]. In these cases, the LAD frequently shows anastomotic connections with the left posterior descending artery (PDA)[2].

The LAD gives some branches along its course[2–4,6,8–12]:

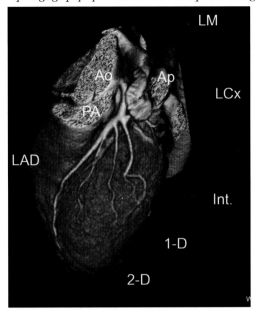

FIGURE 2.7 Anatomical relationships of left main (LM) coronary artery. Ao: aorta; Ap: left atrial appendage; Int.: intermediate artery; LAD: left anterior descending; LCx: circumflex artery; PA: pulmonary artery; 1D and 2D: first and second diagonal branches of the LAD.

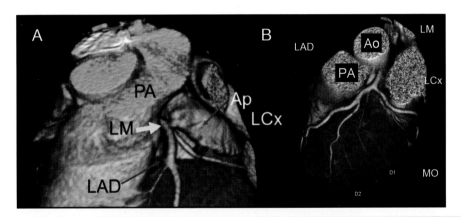

FIGURE 2.8 Anatomical relationships of the proximal segments of the main branches of the left coronary artery. Observe the course of the vessels below the left atrial appendage (Ap) in A, which is adequately displayed when the Ap is removed, in B. Ao: aorta; LAD: left anterior descending; LCx: circumflex artery; LM: left main; MO: marginal obtuse branch of the LCx; PA: pulmonary artery; 1D and 2D: first and second diagonal branches of the LAD.

— *Left conal artery* (Figure 2.5): with an origin in the proximal LAD, it communicates with the right conal artery, with which it constitutes the "arterial ring of Vieussens," along with the *vasa vasorum* of the aorta and pulmonary artery.

— *Right anterior ventricular branches*: usually irrelevant in number and diameter, as the right ventricle is almost exclusively irrigated through the right coronary artery.

— *Left anterior ventricular branches (diagonal arteries)*[13–15] (Figure 2.7): Variable in number, these branches distribute diagonally over the anterior aspect of the left ventricle (Figure 2.12). The origin of the first diagonal artery (Figure 2.5) is used as the anatomical point dividing the middle and distal segments of the LAD. Frequently, one of these diagonal arteries is particulary large and follows a course parallel to the

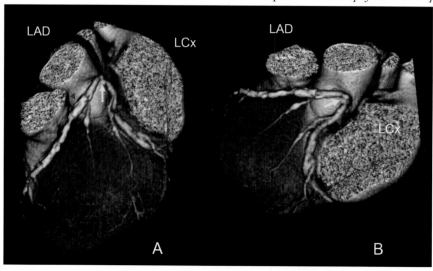

FIGURE 2.9 Left oblique (A) and left lateral (B) views in a case of absent left main (LM) (yellow arrow), with an independent origin of the left anterior descending (LAD) and circumflex (LCx) arteries. Observe the extensive vessel wall calcification.

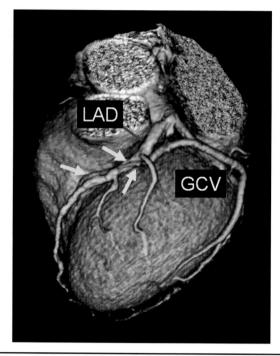

FIGURE 2.10 Relationship between the left anterior descending (LAD) and the great cardiac vein (GCV), showing vessel crossing at their middle course (yellow arrows).

LAD (Figure 2.12D), from which it can be distiguished by the lack of septal branches and the presence of secondary small diagonal branches. In cases where this diagonal artery reaches the obtuse margin of the heart, and from there, the posterior aspect of the left ventricle, it is known as posterolateral artery. The absence of diagonal arteries is extremely rare and, thus, when this is the case in coronary angiography, occlusion of some of these branches can be suspected.

– *Anterior septal branches*: variable in number, these branches arise orthogonally from the LAD and distribute into the anterior two-

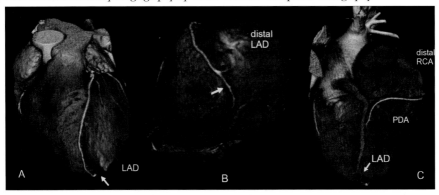

FIGURE 2.11 Recurrent course of the distal segment of the left anterior descending (LAD) artery reaching the interventricular posterior groove. A: anterior view; B: apical view; C: posterior view. PDA: posterior descending artery.

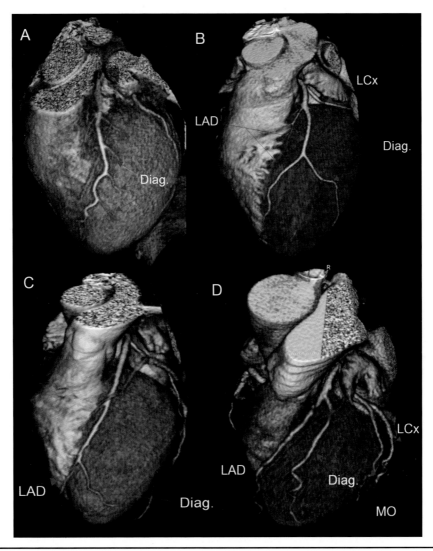

FIGURE 2.12 Normal anatomical variants of diagonal (Diag) branches. A: Multiple small brief branches; B: Single branch emerging from the middle left anterior descending (LAD); C: Single branch emerging from the distal LAD; D: Large vessel coursing parallel to the LAD; LCx: left circumflex; MO: marginal obtuse branch.

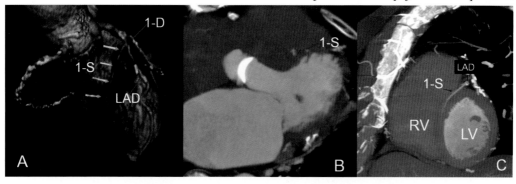

FIGURE 2.13 First septal branch (1-S) of the left anterior descending (LAD). A: The weak contrast opacification of the right heart chambers allows the visualization of the course of 1-S through the interventricular septum; B and C: Maximal Intensity Projection (MIP) images showing transverse (B) and longitudinal (C) sections of 1-S into the septum; LV: left ventricle; RV: right ventricle.

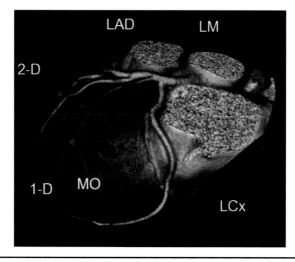

FIGURE 2.14 Left circumflex (LCx) artery ending at the (left) obtuse margin of the heart. LAD: left anterior descending; LM: left main; MO: marginal obtuse; 1D and 2D: first and second diagonal branches.

thirds of the interventricular septum. The first septal branch is usually a well developed vessel (Figure 2.13), its origin being considered as the reference point dividing the proximal and middle portions of the LAD. Rarely, this first septal branch courses closely parallel to the LAD.

2.2.3 Left circumflex (LCx)

LCx artery is also a large vessel, similar in diameter to the LAD, although more variable in terms of length and anatomical distribution[3,4]. The proximal portion of the vessel lies beneath the left atrial appendage and, from there, its course follows the anterior aspect of the left atrioventricular groove, ending at the obtuse

margin of the heart (Figure 2.14). In some cases, the vessel extends to the posterior aspect of the left atrioventricular groove, usually below the coronary venous sinus, ending proximally to the region of the *crux cordis*[2–4]. Finally, in cases of anatomical dominance of the left coronary system, the LCx goes beyond this region and gives the PDA.

The LCx gives origin to different branches during its course[2–4,6,8–12]:

– *Anterior or anterolateral ventricular branches*: when present, these small vessels (Figures 2.15, 2.16A) arise proximally and course parallel to the first diagonal artery. When this artery is absent, it is substituted by these branches.

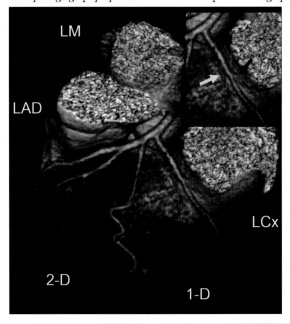

FIGURE 2.15 Left circumflex (LCx) artery, with a small anterolateral branch (yellow arrow) and an atrial branch (black arrow) (see inset at top right). LAD: left anterior descending; LM: left main; 1D and 2D: first and second diagonal branches.

— *Sinusal or sinoatrial branch*[16,17] (Figure 2.16): although usually arising from the right artery, the sinusal branch emerges from the proximal segment of the LCx in 30–35% of individuals, courses around the left atrium, and reaches the sinus node region at the superior vena cava drainage.

— *Atrial arteries* (Figure 2.15): these small vessels are usually located beneath the base of the left atrial appendage or at the posterior aspect of the left atrium.

— *Obtuse marginal branches* (Figure 2.17): usually one or two, their origin is used as a reference dividing the proximal and medial segments of the LCx. These branches are well-developed vessels emerging orthogonally from the LCx and coursing along the left margin of the heart until they reach the apex, where they can communicate with vessels from the LAD.

— *Posterior ventricular branches* (Figures 2.17A, 2.18, 2.19): although the posterior wall of the left ventricle is mostly irrigated by branches from the right PDA, when this vessel is absent, a variable number of these posterior ventricular branches—together with a number of interventricular branches of the LCx—are responsible for the blood supply to this region.

— *Atrioventricular nodal branch*: it arises from the LCx in up to 20% of subjects, particularly in cases of left dominance.

2.2.4 Intermediate coronary artery

In a proportion of individuals, reported as between 25–40%, the LM divides into three branches; in addition to the LAD and the LCx, a third vessel is found, known as median or intermediate artery, arising from the vertex of the angle formed by the two former arteries[4] (Figure 2.20).

Usually a large vessel, the intermediate artery runs over the antero-lateral aspect of the left ventricle, giving septal anterior branches (Figure 2.21) as well as to the anterior papillary muscle. The length of the vessel is variable, although frequently it ends near the obtuse left margin of the heart. Not rarely, however, it reaches the apex or even the inferior aspect of the left ventricle.

In those cases with a largely developed intermediate artery, the diagonal and obtuse marginal arteries are, accordingly, smaller vessels.

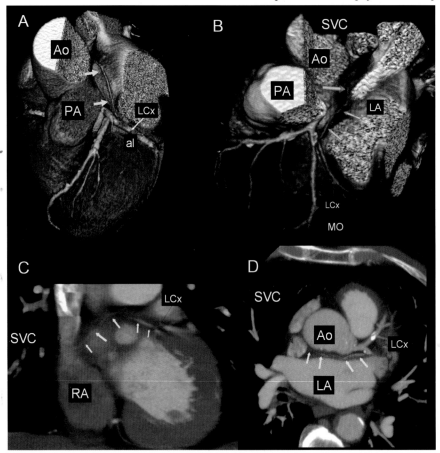

FIGURE 2.16 Left circumflex (LCx) artery. A: Anterior view showing an anterolateral (al) branch (red arrow) and a sinus branch (yellow arrows); B: Cranial view also displaying the sinus branch (yellow arrows); C: MPR on an oblique view with volume render, and; D: Axial slice with MIP, both showing the sinus branch of the LCx and its course towards the region of the superior vena cava (SVC); Ao: aorta; LA: left atrium; MO: marginal obtuse branch; PA: pulmonary artery; RA: right atrium.

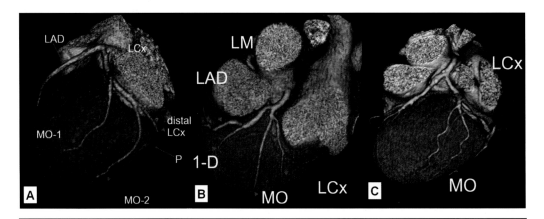

FIGURE 2.17 Anatomy of marginal obtuse (MO) branches. A: Two MO branches are seen (1 and 2) and, also, a posterior branch irrigating the posterior aspect of the left ventricle; B: Occasionally, only a single MO branch is present which arises early from the left circumflex (LCx) and is frequently larger than the LCx itself; C: Bifurcated MO branch; LAD: left anterior descending; LM: left main; 1D: first diagonal.

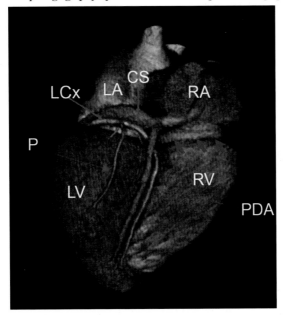

FIGURE 2.18 Anatomical dominance of the left coronary system, with a posterior descending artery (PDA) depending from the left circumflex (LCx); a posterior (P) branch of the LCx is seen irrigating the posterior aspect of the left ventricle (LV) , while the right coronary artery does not reach the inferior aspect of the heart (blue arrows). CS: coronary sinus; LA: left atrium; RA: right atrium; RV: right ventricle.

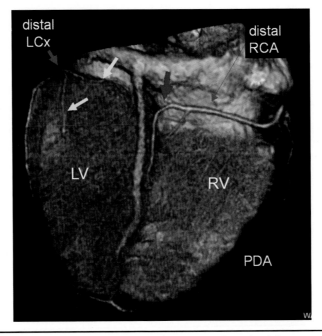

FIGURE 2.19 Anatomical dominance of the right coronary system where the right coronary artery (RCA) gives origin to the posterior descending artery (PDA) but not to posterolateral branches (blue arrow). This myocardial territory depends, in this case, from posterior branches (yellow arrows) emerging from the distal left circumflex (LCx). LV: left ventricle; RV: right ventricle.

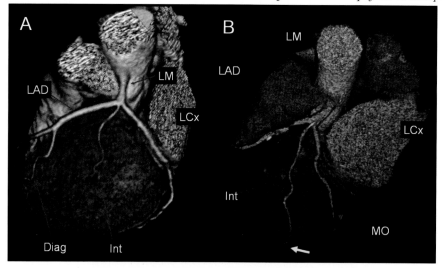

FIGURE 2.20 Intermediate (Int) coronary arteries from two different subjects: in case B, the vessel is large, reaching the left margin of the heart (yellow arrow). Diag: diagonal branch; LAD: left anterior descending; LCx: circumflex artery; LM: left main; MO: marginal obtuse branch.

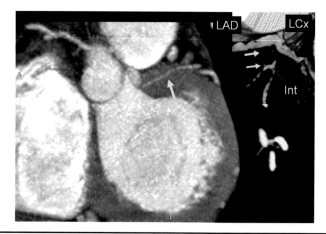

FIGURE 2.21 Example of septal branch originated from one of the bifurcating branches of an intermediate (Int) artery (yellow arrows, at the inset, top right) with an intramyocardial course through the anteroseptal wall (arrow on the large panel). LAD: left anterior descending; LCx: circumflex artery.

2.3 Right Coronary Artery (RCA)

The RCA supplies the blood flow for the right atria and ventricle and, when dominant, also for a variable extension of the posterior aspect of the left ventricle.

Originated in the right coronary sinus, the proximal segment of the RCA courses closely to the right atrial appendage and is then located on the anterior aspect of the right atrioventricular groove, where it is embedded in adipose tissue (Figure 2.22). At its medial segment, the RCA rounds the right acute margin of the heart and through the posterior aspect of the right atrioventricular groove, it reaches the region of the *crux cordis*[2–4,6,8] (Figure 2.23).

There are variants of this anatomical distribution: in 10% of individuals the RCA ends at the level of the acute margin of the heart (Figure 2.24), or between this region and the *crux cordis*; in 60% the RCA extends beyond the *crux cordis* and reaches the inferior wall of the left ventricle (Figure 2.23A), where it shows connections with the distal LCx artery; finally, in 20% of subjects the vessel arrives

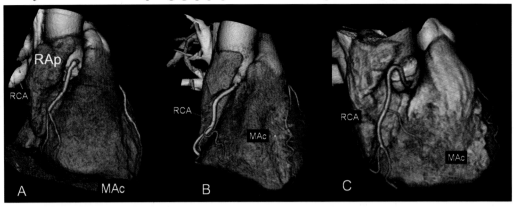

FIGURE 2.22 Anatomy of the right coronary artery (RCA). A: Proximal and middle segments of the vessel coursing in close relationship with the right atrial appendage (RAp) and giving origin to the marginal acute branch (MAc); B: Example of a tortuous MAc; C: Early bifurcation of the RCA at its middle segment (blue arrows).

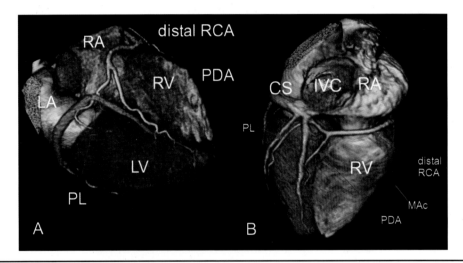

FIGURE 2.23 Anatomy of the distal right coronary artery (RCA). A: Bifurcation of the vessel near the region of the *crux cordis* into a posterior descending artery (PDA) and a posterolateral (PL) branch; B: Example of a long PL branch reaching the left margin of the heart; a marginal acute (MAc) artery is also seen over the right margin; CS: coronary sinus; IVC: inferior vena cava; LA: left atrium; LV: left ventricle; RA: right atrium; RV: right ventricle.

to the left cardiac margin, irrigating the area corresponding to the LCx (Figure 2.23B).

The RCA gives different branches along its course[2–4,6,8–12]:

–　*Right conal branch*: as mentioned earlier, in up to 36% of individuals, this vessel shows an origin in the anterior aspect of the right coronary sinus, independent from the one of the RCA (Figure 2.4). Usually a small vessel, the right conal branch may occasionally be large, supplying an extense portion of the right ventricle, in which case, the RCA appears less developed (Figure 2.25). As described above, the right and left conal

branches are connected, constituting the "arterial ring of Vieussens."

–　*Sinus node branch*[16,17] (Figure 2.26): this vessel originates from the RCA in more than 50% of individuals, usually arising from the most proximal portion of the RCA or, rarely, from its middle or even distal segment. The sinus node branch courses over the base of the right atrial appendage, ending at the drainage of the superior vena cava into the right atrium.

–　*Atrial branches*: variable in number and size, these branches are distributed over the anterolateral aspect of the right atrium, although a posterior branch also does exist,

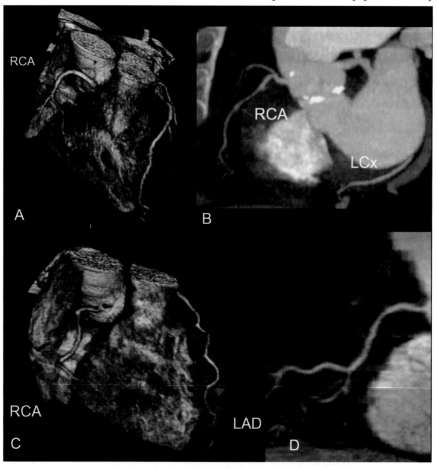

FIGURE 2.24

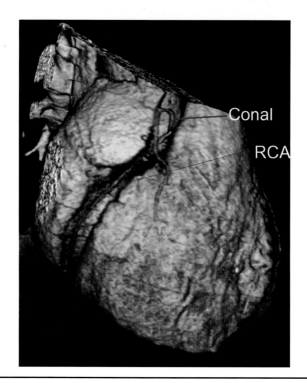

FIGURE 2.25

F. 2.24. Anatomical dominance of the left coronary system with poorly developed right coronary artery (RCA), not reaching the right margin of the heart. Two cases are presented (A-B and C-D) with 3D volume rendering images (left panels) and curved MPR (right panels). LAD: left anterior descending; LCx: circumflex artery.

F. 2.25. Right conal artery in a case with a relatively narrow right coronary artery (RCA).

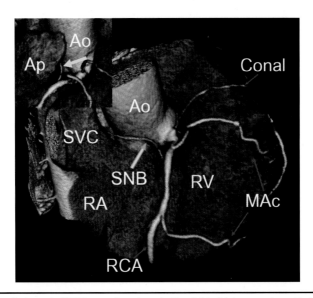

FIGURE 2.26 Sinus node branch (SNB) coursing close to the right atrial appendage (Ap) (see inset, at top left) and ending near the region of drainage of the superior vena cava (SVC). Ao: aorta; MAc: marginal acute branch; RA; right atrium; RV: right ventricle.

supplying both atria or the posterior left atrium exclusively.

- *Acute marginal branch*: this anterior right ventricular branch is usually a well-developed vessel, coursing over the right ventricular free wall (Figure 2.27), near the right acute margin of the heart, and reaching the region of the apex in most individuals. Not infrequently, one or two additional marginal branches are seen emerging from the RCA and running parallel to the acute marginal branch, which is, however, the larger vessel (Figure 2.28).

- *Posterior right ventricular branches*: these are small vessels—not always present—arising from the distal RCA, and irrigating the inferior aspect of the right ventricle (Figure 2.29). Their degree of development is inverse to that of the acute marginal branch, which occasionally distributes over the same region (Figure 2.30).

- *Interventricular posterior branch (or right PDA)*: this artery is a branch of the RCA in up to 90% of individuals, arising from the *crux cordis*, or the region where both

posterior atrioventricular grooves meet with the posterior interventricular groove. In nearly 70% of subjects, the right PDA is a single branch (Figure 2.23A) coursing along the posterior interventricular groove, ending next to the most distal recurrent branch of the LAD, in the region of the apex. In the remaining 30% of cases, 2 or 3 smaller branches are present, coursing in parallel at both sides of the interventricular groove (Figure 2.31). In some cases, the right PDA originates from the RCA at some point between the right acute cardiac margin and the *crux cordis*, coursing diagonally over the inferior aspect of the right ventricle (Figure 2.32). The PDA irrigates the posterior aspect of both ventricles, also giving small posterior septal branches in those cases when the vessel courses along the posterior interventricular groove. These branches penetrate into the posterior septum in a lesser extention than the anterior ones and are usually lacking at the apical region. The first of these posterior septal branches is frequently a well-developed vessel emerging

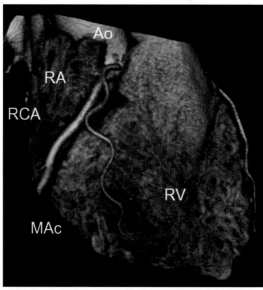

FIGURE 2.27 Independent origin of a marginal acute (MAc) branch from the aorta (Ao) (blue arrow). RA: right atrium; RCA: right coronary artery; RV: right ventricle.

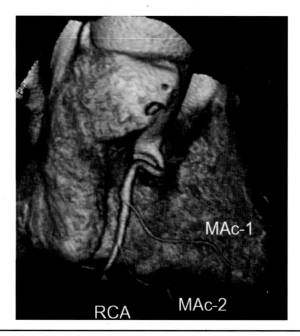

FIGURE 2.28 Marginal acute (MAc-1, MAc-2) branches of the right coronary artery (RCA), which shows a tortuous course at its proximal segment (blue arrow). Observe the long course of the MAc-1, reaching the cardiac apex.

at the level of the *crux cordis*, irrigating the atrioventricular node (Figure 2.33).

– *Right posterobasal or posterolateral arteries*: widely variable in number, size, and distribution pattern, these vessels usually course over the inferior aspect of the left ventricle (Figure 2.34).

2.4 Pattern of Dominance of the Coronary Arteries

The term "dominant" is widely used in the clinical setting as referred to the coronary artery that reaches the crux cordis and gives origin to

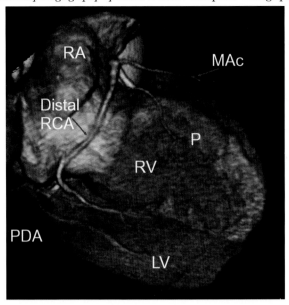

FIGURE 2.29 Posterior right ventricular branch (P). MAc: marginal acute branch; LV: left ventricle; PDA; posterior descending artery; RA: right atrium; RCA: right coronary artery; RV: right ventricle.

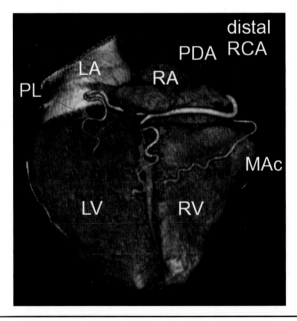

FIGURE 2.30 Marginal acute (MAc) branch of the right coronary artery (RCA) extending into the inferior aspect of the right ventricle similarly to the posterior right ventricular branch (see Figure 2.29). LA: left atrium; LV: left ventricle; PDA: posterior descending artery; PL: posterolateral branch; RA: right atrium; RV: right ventricle.

the PDA. However, this expression can falsely lead to the assumption that a particular coronary artery is responsible for the irrigation of most of the ventricular myocardial mass, while it is the left coronary artery (whether or not "dominant"), which actually supplies the largest amount of ventricular myocardium in most normal hearts[2–4,18].

Anatomical macroscopic exams show a relatively constant pattern of distribution of the

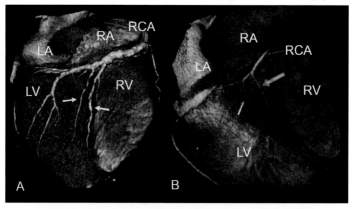

FIGURE 2.31 Examples of posterior descending arteries (PDA): sometimes not a single vessel, but consisting of two or more branches (arrows) of large (A) or small (B) diameter, arising from the distal right coronary artery (RCA). LA: left atrium; LV: left ventricle; RA: right atrium; RV: right ventricle.

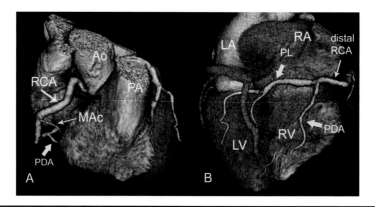

FIGURE 2.32 Anterior (A) and posterior (B) views from a subject with a posterior descending artery (PDA) originating from the right coronary artery (RCA) proximally to the region of the *crux cordis*, presenting with a diagonal course over the inferior wall of the right ventricle. Ao: aorta; MAc: marginal acute branch; LA: left atrium; LV: left ventricle; PA: pulmonary artery; RA: right atrium; RV: right ventricle.

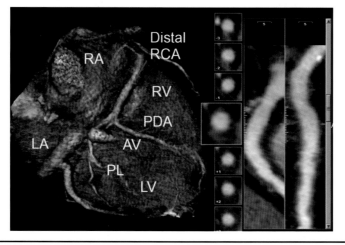

FIGURE 2.33 Atrioventricular (AV) node artery (blue arrow) originating from the right coronary artery (RCA) at the level of the *crux cordis*. LA: left atrium; LV: left ventricle; PDA: posterior descending artery; PL: posterolateral branch; RA: right atrium; RV: right ventricle.

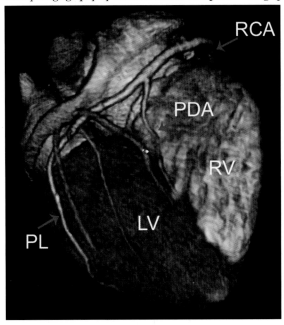

FIGURE 2.34 Large posterolateral branch (PL) from the right coronary artery (RCA) reaching the left margin of the heart. LV: left ventricle; PDA: posterior descending artery; RV: right ventricle.

coronary circulation at the level of the anterior aspect of the heart, in contrast with the inferior aspect, where there is more variability, as blood supply is provided by the distal RCA and LCx, both with a degree of development which is complementary to each other.

Three patterns of anatomical coronary artery dominance can be distiguished (Baroldi and Scomazzoni, 1965):

— *Type I* (77% of individuals): in this case, the RCA gives origin to the PDA, and in turn, may end up with different patterns: (a) at the posterior interventricular groove, rarely with branching vessels for the left ventricle (5%) (Figure 2.19); (b) providing distinctive medium-sized branches for a portion of the inferior aspect of the left ventricle (55%) (Figure 2.23A); and (c) with large branches for most of the inferior aspect of the left ventricle, reaching the left cardiac margin (17%) (Figure 2.23B).
— *Type II* (8%): in this case, the PDA is a branch of the LCx, appearing either as a single or a ramified vessel (Figures 2.18, 2.35).
— *Type III* (*"balanced" circulation*) (15%): in this case there are two PDA, one provided for each vessel (RCA and LCx), coursing in parallel to the posterior interventricular groove (Figure 2.36). In this pattern, the

apex of the heart and the inferior aspect of the interventricular septum are irrigated by the left coronary artery.

A knowledge of these patterns of anatomic dominance is fundamental for an appropriate assessment of a coronary angiography, where a relatively frequent cause of concern is the distinction between a branch occlusion and a normal anatomical pattern of the PDA.

2.5 Congenital Anomalies of the Coronary Arteries

Congenital anomalies of the coronary arteries comprise a number of entities where features different from those considered as defining normalcy are present[19] (Table 2.1).

Despite the large number of reported anomalies[20–22] (Table 2.2), congenital anomalies of coronary arteries are present with low prevalence rates; lower than 3% of all congenital heart diseases, and less than 1% of the general population[23]. Congenital anomalies of coronary arteries may be present in the absence of other structural heart disease[24–26] or, more frequently, they are found in patients with D-transposition of the great vessels[27–29]

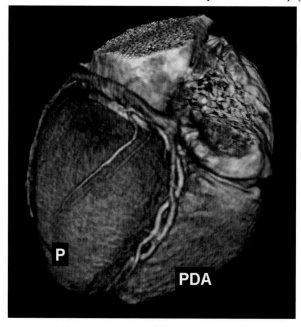

FIGURE 2.35 Posterior descending artery (PDA) originating from the circumflex artery in a subject with "left dominance." P: posterior ventricular branch.

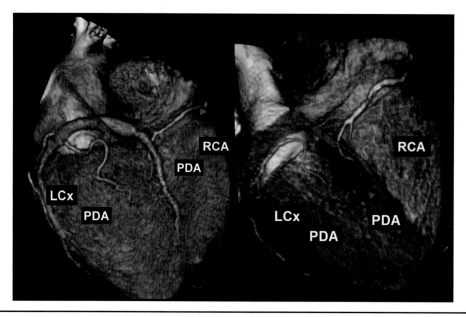

FIGURE 2.36 Two different subjects with a balanced coronary circulation pattern: both the right coronary artery (RCA) and the left circumflex artery (LCx) give origin to a posterior descending artery (PDA) from their own.

(Figure 2.37), Fallot's tetralogy, pulmonary atresia with ventricular septal defect, or, in general, in patients with chromosomic abnormalities (trisomy 18)[28,30]. Not rarely, they are incidental findings in coronary angiographies performed due to symptoms not related with these abnormalities.

Congenital anomalies of the coronary arteries may be the cause of myocardial ischemia and even sudden death[31]. For this reason, it is clinically important to recognize two different types of these anomalies[32], depending on whether or not they are able to produce myocardial ischemia.

Table 2.1 Normal coronary artery anatomical features and corresponding congenital anomalies (adapted from Trivellato[19]).

	Normal	Abnormal
• Coronary *ostia*	Two	One
• Course of main trunks	Epicardial	Intramural
• Course of RCA	Right AV groove	Left side (partially)
• Course of LCA	Left AV and interventricular anterior grooves	Right side (partially)
• PDA origin	RCA or LCx	LAD
• Coronary artery drainage	Capillary bed	Other

Table 2.2 Congenital coronary artery abnormalities (adapted from Angelini[20–22]).

A. Anomalies of the origin and course of vessels
   1. Absent left main trunk
   2. Anomalous location of a coronary *ostium* within the proper coronary sinus
   3. Anomalous location of a coronary *ostium* at places other than the normal coronary sinuses
      a. Right posterior aortic sinus
      b. Thoracic aorta, supraortic vessels, and their branches
      c. Left and right ventricle
      d. Pulmonary artery (Bland-White-Garland syndrome, in case of LCA)
   4. RCA/LCA arising from the contrary sinus, with anomalous course:
      a. Posterior atrioventricular groove or retrocardiac
      b. Retroaortic
      c. Between aorta and pulmonary artery
      d. Intraseptal
      e. Anterior to pulmonary outflow or precardiac
      f. Posteroanterior interventricular groove
   5. Single coronary artery (40% associated to other congenital heart diseases)
B. Anomalies of intrinsic coronary arterial anatomy
   1. Congenital ostial stenosis or atresia
   2. Absent coronary artery
   3. Coronary hypoplasia
   4. Intramural coronary artery (muscular bridge)
   5. Subendocardial coronary course
   6. Coronary crossing
   7. Anomalous origin of PDA from a branch of the LAD or from a septal penetrating branch
   8. Absent LAD or PDA
   9. Ectopic origin of first septal branch
C. Anomalies of coronary drainage
   1. Inadequate arteriolar/capillary ramifications
   2. Fistulas from RCA or LCA
D. Anomalous collateral vessels

2.5.1 Anomalies relatable to myocardial ischemia

In most of these anomalies, a segment of a coronary artery is seen to course abnormally between the wall of the aortic root and that of the main pulmonary artery[33–36] (Figures 2.38–2.40). This situation may cause exertional myocardial ischemia due to enlargement of the great vessels, secondary to transiently increased flow[32]. Also, in cases of abnormal coronary artery course around the anterior aspect of the pulmonary artery (Figure 2.41), ischemia may be present in those situations of enlargement of the right ventricular outflow tract, as in pulmonary hypertension[37,38].

Abnormal origin of coronary arteries from the pulmonary artery, either the LCA (Bland-White-Garland syndrome)[39,40] or the RCA, is also an obvious cause of myocardial ischemia.

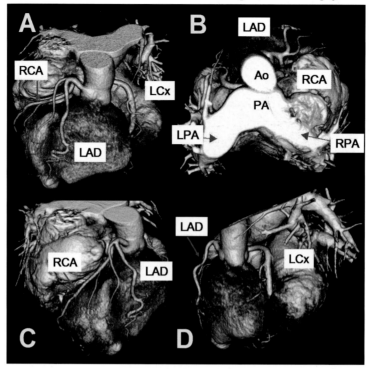

FIGURE 2.37

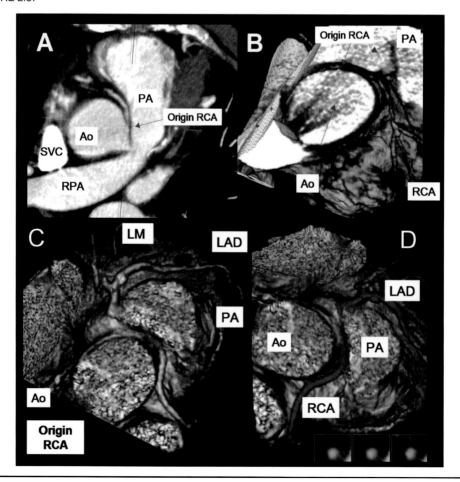

FIGURE 2.38

F. 2.37.   Patient with transposition of the great arteries and an associated anomaly of the origin and course of the coronary arteries. A (anterior view): The left anterior descending (LAD) is seen at the anterior interventricular groove; B (cranial view) and C (right anterior oblique view): The LAD and the right coronary artery (RCA) arise from a common trunk; D (left anterior oblique view): The circumflex artery (LCx) emerges independently from the posterior sinus of Valsalva; Ao: aorta; LPA: left pulmonary artery; PA: main pulmonary artery; RPA: right pulmonary artery.

F. 2.38.   Anomalous origin of the right coronary artery (RCA), emerging from the left coronary sinus of Valsalva and following an interarterial course between the aorta (Ao) and the pulmonary artery (PA) from two different patients (A,B and C,D). A: Axial oblique MPR; B-D: 3D volume rendering reconstructions (cranial view); LAD: left anterior descending; LM: left main trunk; RPA: right pulmonary artery; SVC: superior vena cava.

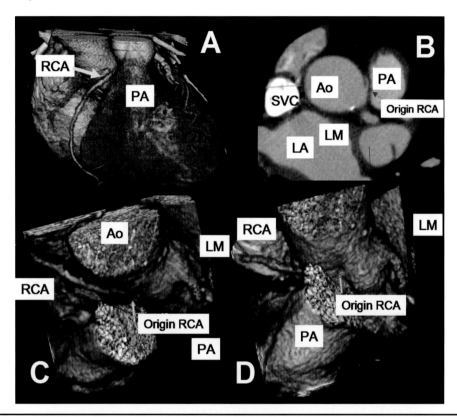

FIGURE 2.39 Anomalous origin of the right coronary artery (RCA) emerging from the left sinus of Valsalva, viewed from 3D volume rendering images (A, C, D) and oblique MPR (B), all from the same patient. Ao: aorta; LA: left atrium; LM: left main; PA: pulmonary artery; SVC: superior vena cava.

2.5.2 Anomalies not leading to myocardial ischemia

Some of the congenital coronary anomalies are not related to myocardial ischemia and are detected incidentally. However, their knowledge is important for two reasons, particularly when non-coronary cardiac surgery is planned to prevent inadvertent damage of the aberrant coronary vessel, and to appropriately guide the coronary artery cannulation[25,37,41–43].

These coronary anomalies have been detected in 0.5–1% of invasive coronary angiographies, although it is not always feasible to describe at angiography the exact course of the abnormal artery in relation to the great vessels[44]. MDCT has shown better diagnostic accuracy in this aspect, provided its ability to present 3D reconstructed images[45–47].

The most frequently found types of coronary anomalies are the following:

Origin of the LCx from the right coronary sinus or RCA (Figures 2.42–2.44): It is the most frequent anomaly in this group (0.67% of diagnostic invasive coronary angiograms)[32,48] and it seems to be more frequent in cases of congenital stenosis of the aortic valve[38,43]. The LCx is seen emerging posteriorly to the RCA, and then following a course inferior and

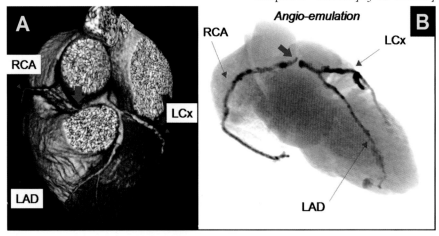

FIGURE 2.40 Anomalous origin of the right coronary artery (RCA) from the left sinus of Valsalva (blue arrows). A: 3D volume rendering; B: Postprocessed images emulating an angiography; LAD: left anterior descending. LCx: circumflex artery.

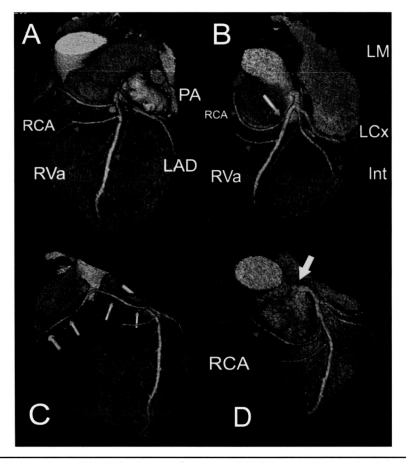

FIGURE 2.41 Anomalous origin of the right coronary artery (RCA) from the left anterior descending (LAD) coronary artery. These 3D volume rendering images correspond to the same patient, showing the origin of the RCA (A and B: yellow arrow) and the course of the vessel around the anterior aspect of the pulmonary valve ring, reaching its normal position at the right atrioventricular groove (C: yellow arrows). Distally to the abnormal origin of the RCA, the LAD gives a second abnormal branch for the right ventricle (RVa). Observe that the entire coronary arterial supply comes from a single trunk (D: yellow arrow). Int: Intermediate artery; LCx: left circumflex; LM: left main trunk.

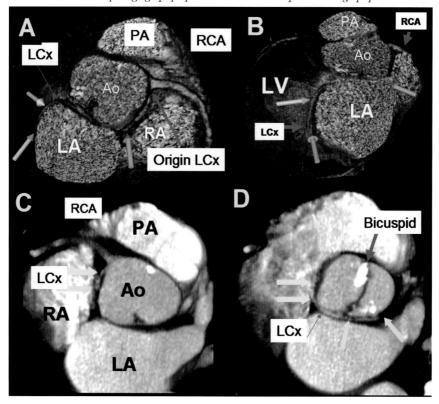

FIGURE 2.42 Patient with anomalous origin of the left circumflex artery (LCx) from the right coronary sinus of Valsalva (panels A and C), with a retroaortic course to the left atrioventricular groove (B and D). Observe the presence of a bicuspid aortic valve (panel D). Ao: aorta; LA: left atrium; LV: left ventricle; PA: pulmonary artery; RA: right atrium; RCA: right coronary artery.

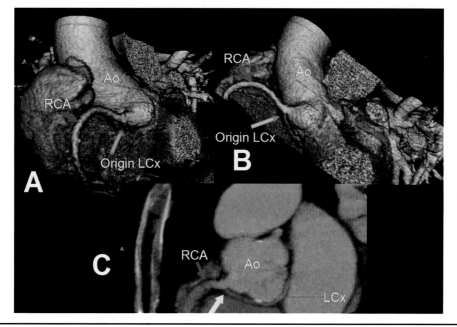

FIGURE 2.43 Patient with anomalous origin of the left circumflex artery (LCx) from the right coronary artery (RCA) (panels A and B). Observe the marked angulation of the origin of the LCx from the RCA and its retroaortic course to reach the left atrioventricular groove (panel C). Ao: Aorta.

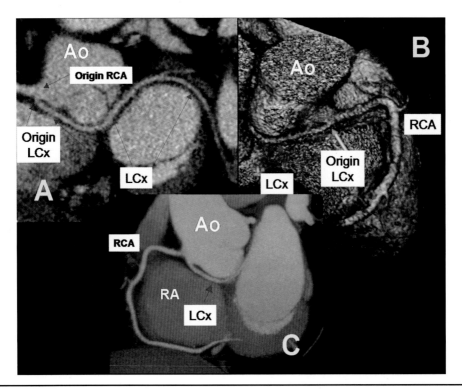

FIGURE 2.44

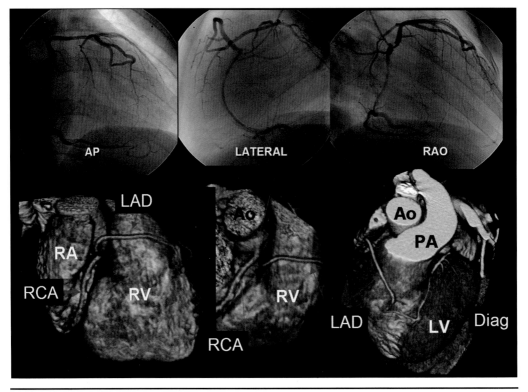

FIGURE 2.45

F. 2.44.   Examples of anomalous origin of the left circumflex artery (LCx) from the right coronary artery (RCA) (panel A: curved MPR and panel B: 3D volume rendering-, from the same patient) and directly from the right coronary sinus of Valsalva (panel C: MIP image). Ao: Aorta. RA: right atrium.

F. 2.45.   Patient with anomalous origin of the left anterior descending (LAD). Although the abnormal origin and course of the arteries is already evident on the images from the invasive angiography (top panels), the actual origin of the LAD (from the right coronary artery (RCA) or directly from the sinus of Valsalva) and their course in relation to the great vessels can only be discerned from the MDCT angiography (bottom panels). Observe the origin of the LAD from the RCA and its course over the anterior aspect of the right ventricular outflow tract, reaching the anterior interventricular groove. Ao: aorta; AP: anteroposterior; Diag: diagonal artery; LV: left ventricle; PA: pulmonary artery; RA: right atrium; RAO: right anterior oblique; RV: right ventricle.

posterior to the aortic root, reaching the left atrioventricular groove. Very rare in this case is a course of the LCx between the walls of the great vessels.

Origin of the LAD in the RCA (Figure 2.45): This anomaly is present in 4–5% of patients with tetralogy of Fallot or pulmonary atresia with ventricular septal defect[25]. The LAD frequently shows a course anterior to the infundibular portion of the right ventricle, usually not leading to myocardial ischemia, which has potential implications in the case of surgical correction.

References

1. National Heart, Lung, and Blood Institute Coronary Artery Surgery Study. A multicenter comparison of the effects of randomized medical and surgical treatment of mildly symptomatic patients with coronary artery disease, and a registry of consecutive patients undergoing coronary angiography. Circulation 1981, 63, I1–81.

2. *Gray's Anatomy, 38th ed.* New York: Churchill Livingstone, 1995.

3. Petit, M., and J. Reig. *Arterias Coronarias: Aspectos Anatomo-clínicos, 1st ed.* Barcelona: Masson-Salvat, 1993.

4. Reig, J. Anatomical variations of the coronary arteries: I. The most frequent variations. *Eur J Anat*, 2003, 7 (Suppl 1), 29–41.

5. Reig, J., and M. Petit. Main trunk of the left coronary artery: anatomic study of the parameters of clinical interest. *Clin Anat*, 2004, 17, 6–13.

6. Testut, L., and A. Latarjet. *Tratado de Anatomía Humana, 9th ed.* Barcelona: Salvat, 1986.

7. Perlmutt, L.M., M.E. Jay, and D.C. Levin. Variations in the blood supply of the left ventricular apex. *Invest Radiol*, 1983, 18, 138–40.

8. Orts, L.F. *Anatomía Humana, 6th ed.* Barcelona: Científico-Médica, 1986.

9. Rohen, J.W., and Ch. Yokochi. *Atlas fotográfico de Anatomía Humana, 1st ed.* Barcelona: Doyma, 1986.

10. Sobotta, J. *Atlas de Anatomía, 18th ed.* Madrid: Medicina Panamericana, 1983.

11. Netter, F.H. *Atlas de Anatomía Humana, 2nd ed.* New Jersey: Masson-Novartis, 1999.

12. Cavalcanti, J.S., et al. Anatomic variations of the coronary arteries. *Arq Bras Cardiol*, 1995, 65, 489–92.

13. Levin, D.C., et al. Anatomic variations of the left coronary arteries supplying the anterolateral aspect of the left ventricle: Possible explanation for the "unexplained" anterior aneurysm. *Invest Radiol*, 1982, 17, 458–62.

14. Spindola-Franco, H., R. Grose, and N. Solomon. Dual left anterior descending coronary artery: angiographic description of important variants and surgical implications. *Am Heart J*, 1983, 105, 445–55.

15. Chiurlia, E., et al. Type IV dual left anterior descending coronary artery evaluated using multislice computed tomography: anatomy of a rare coronary anomaly. *Ital Heart J*, 2003, 4, 900–1.

16. Ovcina, F., and D. Cemerlic. Clinical importance of intramural blood vessels in the sino-atrial segment of the conducting system of the heart. *Surg Radiol Anat*, 1997, 19, 359–63.

17. Kyriakidis, M., et al. A clinical angiographic study of the arterial blood supply to the sinus node. *Chest*, 1988, 94, 1054–7.

18. Gorlin, R. Coronary anatomy. *Major Probl Intern Med*, 1976, 11, 40–58.

19. Trivellato, M., P. Angelini, and R.D. Leachman. Variations in coronary artery anatomy: Normal versus abnormal. *Cardiovasc Dis*, 1980, 7, 357–70.

20. Angelini, P. Normal and anomalous coronary arteries: definitions and classification. *Am Heart J*, 1989, 117, 418–34.

21. Angelini, P., V.D. Fairchild, eds. *Coronary Artery Anomalies: A Comprehensive Approach*. Philadelphia: Lippincott, Williams & Wilkins, 1999.

22. Angelini, P. Coronary artery anomalies–current clinical issues: definitions, classification, incidence, clinical relevance, and treatment guidelines. *Tex Heart Inst J*, 2002, 29, 271–8.

23. Reig, J. Anatomical variations in the coronary arteries.II. Less prevalent variations: Coronary anomalies. *Eur J Anat*, 2004, 8, 39–53.

24. Roberts, W.C. Major anomalies of coronary arterial origin seen in adulthood. *Am Heart J*, 1986, 111, 941–63.

25. Brotons, C. Anomalías coronarias en edad pediátrica. *Anales de Cirugía Cardíaca y Vascular*, 2003, 9, 190–2.

26. Click, R.L., et al. Anomalous coronary arteries: Location, degree of atherosclerosis and effect on survival—a report from the Coronary Artery Surgery Study. *J Am Coll Cardiol*, 1989, 12, 531–7.

27. Ismat, F.A., et al. Coronary anatomy in congenitally corrected transposition of the great arteries. *Int J Cardiol*, 2002, 86, 207–16.

28. Mawson, J.B. Congenital heart defects and coronary anatomy. *Tex Heart Inst J*, 2002, 29, 279–89.

29. Girona, J., et al. Influence of coronary anatomy on the anatomic repair of transposition of great arteries. *Rev Esp Cardiol*, 1996, 49, 451–6.

30. Li, J., et al. Coronary arterial anatomy in tetralogy of Fallot: morphological and clinical correlations. *Heart*, 1998, 80, 174–83.

31. Cheitlin, M.D., C.M. DeCastro, and H.A. McAllister. Sudden death as a complication of anomalous left coronary origin from the anterior sinus of Valsalva, a not-so-minor congenital anomaly. *Circulation*, 1974, 50, 780–7.

32. Braunwald, E., D.P. Zipes, and P. Libby. *Heart Disease: a textbook of cardiovascular Medicine, 6th ed*. Philadelphia: WB Saunders, 2001.

33. Kragel, A.H., and W.C. Robers. Anomalous origin of either the right or left main coronary artery from the aorta with subsequent coursing between aorta and pulmonary trunk: Analysis of 32 necropsy cases. *Am J Cardiol*, 1988, 62, 771–7.

34. Roberts, W.C., R.J. Siegel, and D.P. Zipes. Origin of the right coronary arterial from the left sinus of Valsalva and its functional consequences: Analysis of 10 necropsy patients. *Am J Cardiol*, 1982, 49, 863–8.

35. Kelley, M.J., S. Wolfson, and R. Marshall. Single coronary artery from the right sinus of Valsalva: angiography, anatomy, and clinical significance. *Am J Roentgenol*, 1977, 128, 257–62.

36. Liberthson, R.R., R.E. Dinsmore, and J.T. Fallon. Aberrant coronary artery origin from the aorta: Report of 18 patients, review of literature and delineation of natural history and management. *Circulation*, 1979, 59, 748–54.

37. Kimbiris, D., et al. Anomalous aortic origin of coronary arteries. *Circulation*, 1978, 58, 606–15.

38. Schoepf, U.J. *CT of the heart*. New Jersey: Humana Press, 2005.

39. Tyrrell, M.J., et al. Anomalous left coronary artery from the pulmonary artery: effect of coronary anatomy on clinical course. *Angiology*, 1987, 38, 833–40.

40. Pfannschmidt, J., H. Ruskowski, and E.R. de Vivie. Bland-White-Garland syndrome. Clinical aspects, diagnosis, therapy. *Klin Padiatr*, 1992, 204, 328–34.

41. Gil-Jaurena, J.M. Patología del corazón izquierdo. Anomalías coronarias (aspectos quirúrgicos). *Anales de Cirugía Cardíaca y Vascular*, 2003, 9, 194–6.

42. Kirklin, J.W., and B.G. Barratt-Boyes. *Congenital anomalies of the coronary arteries in Cardiac Surgery, 2nd ed*. New York: Churchill Livingstone, 1992.

43. Topaz, O., et al. Anomalous coronary arteries: angiographic findings in 80 patients. *Int J Cardiol*, 1992, 34, 129–38.

44. Deibler, A.R., et al. Imaging of congenital coronary anomalies with multislice computed tomography. *Mayo Clin Proc*, 2004, 79, 1017–23.

45. van Ooijen, P.M., et al. Detection, visualization and evaluation of anomalous coronary anatomy on 16-slice multidetector-row CT. *Eur Radiol*, 2004, 14, 2163–71.

46. Schmid, M., et al. Visualization of coronary artery anomalies by contrast-enhanced multi-detector row spiral computed tomography. *Int J Cardiol*, 2005 (article in press) doi: 00.1016/j.ijcard. 2005.08.027.

47. Memisoglu, E., et al. Congenital coronary anomalies in adults: comparison of anatomic course visualization by catheter angiography and electron beam CT. *Catheter Cardiovasc Interv*, 2005, 66, 34–42.

48. Page, H.L. Jr., et al. Anomalous origin of the left circumflex coronary artery: Recognition, angiographic demonstration and clinical significance. *Circulation*, 1974, 50, 768–73.

3

3.1 Introduction

Coronary artery calcium (CAC) is an excellent marker of the process of atherosclerosis, as it is present almost exclusively in atherosclerotic plaques of the vessel wall, its amount correlating with the burden of the disease[1]. However, its role in the development of atherosclerotic coronary plaques is not well-defined at present, and because CAC is considered as a marker of the plaque burden, and not a risk factor in itself, its relation with coronary risk has been largely debated[2].

CAC is found extensively in advanced lesions (Figure 3.1), but it may also be present in small amounts in early atherosclerotic lesions already developed on the second or third decades of life (Figure 3.2). The significance of small calcifications in lipid-rich plaques is unclear, as they may be associated with instability[3], while calcification in more advanced lesions may be a stabilizing factor[4]. The number of CAC increases with age, although the rate of progression of CAC in adulthood has been related to the amount of coronary risk factors present earlier in life. In consequence, the prevalence of measurable CAC is lower for people with less risk factors in their youth[5].

In asymptomatic population studies it has been observed that CAC is present in 50% of persons 40 to 49 years old and 80% of those 60 to 69 years old[6]. The incidence of coronary events for these groups of age, however, is far less than it would be anticipated by these figures[7]. Conversely, plaque rupture and acute coronary syndrome can occur in a soft plaque without any calcification, a condition that can occur particularly in young people with a smoking habit[8]. In summary, and according to these observations, the prevalence of CAC correlates better with the presence of atherosclerotic plaques than with acute coronary events[9]. Nevertheless, it has to be considered that the finding of an increased amount of CAC in an asymptomatic person, as a marker of a developed process of coronary atherosclerosis, does imply the probable coexistence of other lipid-rich and, hence, vulnerable plaques[3]. In fact, it has been reported that in 75% of patients with an unheralded myocardial infarction, the amount of calcium was above the 75 percentile when compared to an age and gender matched cohort[10]. Moreover, in early cardiac fluoroscopy studies, the presence of CAC in

FRANCESC CARRERAS

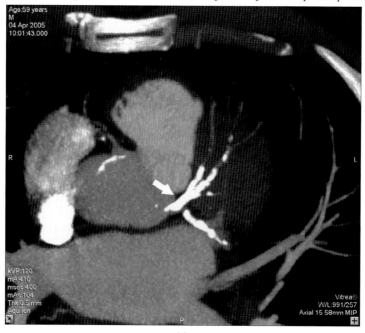

(a)

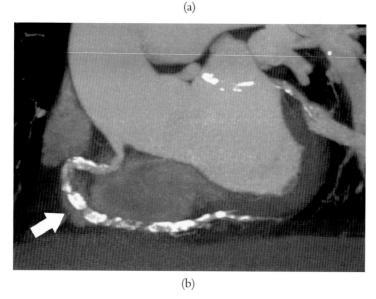

(b)

FIGURE 3.1 Contrast-enhanced maximum intensity projection (MIP) images showing extensive calcification (arrow) of the left main trunk and proximal segments of the left coronary artery (a) and the right coronary artery (b) that prevents an adequate visualization of the vessel wall and lumen.

patients with coronary artery disease had already demonstrated a poorer survival at all follow-up intervals[11].

3.2 CAC Quantification: The Agatston Method

Electron beam computed tomography (EBCT) has proven to be the first noninvasive technique

for the quantification of CAC. Recent technological advances in multidetector computed tomography (MDCT), however, have made this technique superior in the CAC assessment when compared to EBCT[12,13], particularly for the quantitation of the calcium volume, a measurement that strongly depends on image quality[14]. From an epidemiological point of view, data derived from measurements obtained with EBCT on asymptomatic individuals cannot be strictly transferred to those from current

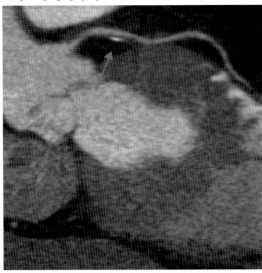

FIGURE 3.2 Contrast-enhanced multiplane reformat reconstruction of the left anterior descending coronary artery, depicting in its proximal segment a predominantly lipid-rich plaque with a small central calcification (arrow).

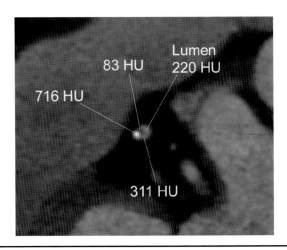

FIGURE 3.3 Contrast-enhanced transverse section of a coronary artery. Values of Hounsfield units are provided for the vessel lumen and every component of the lesion: the higher values (>120 HU) correspond to two plaque areas with different calcium density and contrast media, while the lower values correspond to a soft fibrous area without calcification.

MDCT scanners[15]. Nevertheless, as it has recently been demonstrated that CAC score estimates are concordant with both techniques[16], coronary risk predictions tables from EBCT are applied even though patients are studied by MDCT.

The CAC quantification method adopted for MDCT exams was originally introduced in 1990 by Agatston for EBCT scanners[17], and is based on the maximum x-ray attenuation coefficient, or CT number, measured in Hounsfield units (HU), and the area of calcium deposits. According to this method, densities equal to or greater than 130 HU are considered to correspond to calcium[18] (Figure 3.3). Volume

and mass calculation of the amount of calcium are alternative methods to the Agatston score for the evaluation of the CAC burden. Initial results have shown they are more reproducible and accurate than Agatston scoring[14,19], although additional clinical studies must be performed to confirm these data.

A MDCT CAC scan is acquired within a breath-hold by 2-mm thick ECG-triggered slices of the heart. After the acquisition, the data are processed on a dedicated workstation, which automatically displays the quantities of coronary calcium as equivalent to the Agatston score (volume equivalent and absolute mass) (Figure 3.4).

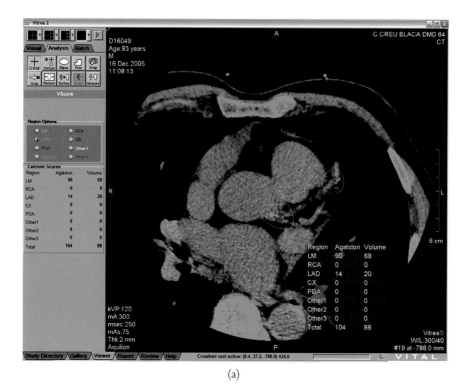

(a)

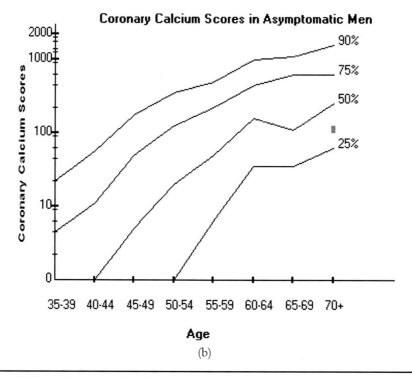

(b)

FIGURE 3.4 (a) Workstation screen displaying a noncontrast enhanced axial image postprocessed with a calcium scoring preset: areas presenting > 130 HU are coloured. A region of interest has been manually drawn, encircling calcified areas at the main trunk and the distal segment of the LAD coronary artery. The volume and calculated Agatston values for the calcified areas are displayed on the screen. (b) Graphics showing the Agatston score (square) for this patient and its position on the percentile curves according to age and gender derived from epidemiological studies on asymptomatic individuals.

3.3 Clinical Implications of CAC

Noninvasive quantification of coronary calcium with EBCT scores has shown to reflect the total atherosclerotic plaque burden in asymptomatic individuals[9], improving risk predictions, particularly in those patients at intermediate risk[20,21]. The identification of high-risk candidates for primary prevention becomes a requirement for preventive medicine. At highest priority are persons without known CHD, whose absolute risk for acute coronary syndromes is as high as that for patients with established CHD[22]. It has been described that a coronary calcium Agatston score of ≥80 has a sensitivity for prediction of coronary events of 0.85 and a specificity of 0.75[23]. Thus, in asymptomatic patients with a prior probability of a coronary event in the intermediate range (>10% but <20% in 10 years), a calcium score ≥80 would yield a post-test probability greater than 2% per year (or >20% per 10 years), which is in the range of patients with previous coronary artery disease. Moreover, it has also been reported that an Agatston score of >160 is related to a 20–35-fold increased risk for a cardiac event[24]. Otherwise, in asymptomatic subjects with a prior probability of a coronary event in the low range, a positive test result with EBCT would not sufficiently increase the likelihood of a coronary event to justify an active intervention[25], this making the test unnecessary in this group of individuals.

There is a growing consensus that "quantitative" risk assessment based on global risk equations, such as those developed by Framingham studies, improves the selection of patients for intensive medical intervention. The use of CAC scores represents an attractive addition to global risk assessment for this purpose, an approach that has been examined in detail by the Prevention V Conference of the American Heart Association, whose conclusions stressed the need to integrate CAC scores with other risk factors in predicting global risk[26]. Recent data from a prospective study confirm the value of CAC scores when combined with Framingham scores to improve risk prediction in asymptomatic individuals, in particular among patients in the intermediate risk category, in whom clinical decision making is most uncertain[27]. In particular, the study demonstrates that a CAC score of more than 300 was associated with a significant increase in coronary heart disease event risk when compared with that determined by the Framingham risk score alone. Furthermore, in these patients, the combination of the CAC score results with noninvasive stress testing results for inducible ischemia would be extremely helpful[28].

Monitoring of CAC progression could be a potential tool for the identification of patients at risk of suffering a myocardial infarction. In a preliminary observational study of 817 subjects with more than one sequential EBCT scan, the patients who suffered a myocardial infarction had a 47% progression of the CAC score, while those who remained event-free progressed about 25% per year[29]. The ultimate question that remains to be answered is whether the slowing of CAC progression with lipid-lowering therapy might save lives and reduce the incidence of myocardial infarction. CAC scores may be used as an end-point for regression therapy, and several observational studies have been published in relation to this subject, although no definite conclusions have been established until now[30,31].

In summary, there is an increasing interest in convincing cardiologists to go beyond the traditional coronary risk factors and, pending the discovery of a simple screening test for the detection of the asymptomatic vulnerable patient, also base the coronary risk prediction in the detection and quantification of CAC as a marker of atherosclerotic disease[32]. Flowcharts suggesting new strategies for the screening of asymptomatic persons, that include CAC score, noninvasive coronary artery imaging, and functional noninvasive stress testing have been suggested by the active groups working on cardiovascular prevention strategies[32]. A proposal for noninvasive coronary risk evaluation of an asymptomatic population based on CAC score is presented in Figure 3.5.

CAC score may be better suited to estimate the risk of unheralded cardiac events in asymptomatic patients than to identify symptomatic patients with ischemic heart disease. Computed tomography CAC screening is a valuable tool that refines risk assessment when used in combination with multivariable statistical models, improving risk prediction for asymptomatic subjects with intermediate pretest probability of cardiovascular events[33] as well as symptomatic patients at low pretest probability[34]. Indiscriminate screening or sequential monitoring of CAC are not recommended in asymptomatic persons,

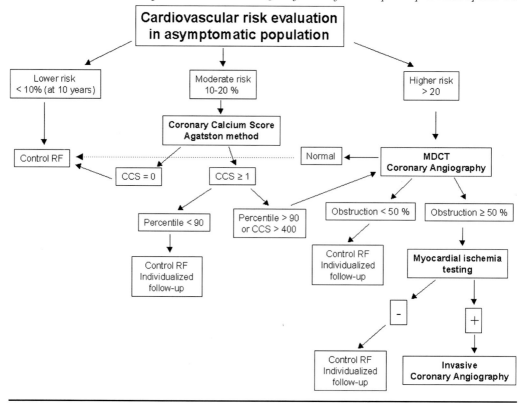

FIGURE 3.5 Proposed algorithm for the detection of coronary artery disease in asymptomatic population, according to the pretest cardiovascular risk, as estimated from the Framingham Heart Study, and MDCT studies.

in which a referral for screening should always be provided by a physician[35].

References

1. Wexler, L., et al. Coronary artery calcification: patophysiology, epidemiology, imaging methods, and clinical implications. *Circulation*, 1996, 94, 1175–92.

2. Pitt, B., and M. Rubenfire. Risk stratification for the detection of preclinical coronary artery disease. *Circulation*, 1999, 99, 2610–2.

3. Schmermund, A., and R. Erbel. Unstable coronary plaque and its relation to coronary calcium. *Circulation*, 2001, 104, 1682–7.

4. Schartl, M., et al. Use of intravascular ultrasound to compare effects of different strategies of lipid-lowering therapy on plaque volume and composition in patients with coronary artery disease. *Circulation*, 2001, 104, 387–92.

5. Daviglus, M.L., et al. Comparison of low risk and higher risk profiles in middle age to fre-

quency and quantity of coronary artery calcium years later. *Am J Cardiol*, 2004, 94, 367–9.

6. Wong, N.D., et al. Coronary calcium and atherosclerosis by ultrafast computed tomography in asymptomatic men and women: relation to age and risk factors. *Am Heart J*, 1994, 127, 422–430.

7. Lloyd-Jones, D.M., et al. Lifetime risk of developing coronary heart disease. *Lancet*, 1999, 353, 89–92.

8. Schmermund, A., et al. Coronary artery calcium in acute coronary syndromes. *Circulation*, 1997, 96, 1461–9.

9. Rumberger, J.A., et al. Coronary artery calcium area by electron-beam computed tomography and coronary atherosclerotic plaque area. A histopathologic correlative study. *Circulation*, 1996, 94, 588.

10. Raggi, P., et al. Identification of patients at increased risk of first unheralded acute myocardial infarction by electron-beam computed tomography. *Circulation*, 2000, 101, 850–5.

11. Margolis, J.R., et al. The diagnostic and prognostic significance of coronary artery calcifica-

tion. A report of 800 cases. *Radiology*, 1980, 137, 609–16.

12. Becker, C.R., et al. Coronary artery calcium measurement: agreement of multirow detector and electron beam CT. *Am J Roentgenol*, 2001, 176, 1295–8.

13. Becker, C.R., et al. CT measurement of coronary calcium mass: impact on global cardiac risk assessment. *Eur Radiol*, 2005, 15, 96–101.

14. Yoon, H.C., et al. Coronary artery calcium: alternate methods for accurate and reproducible quantitation. *Acad Radiol*, 1997, 4, 666–73.

15. Wintersperger, B.J., and K. Nikolau. Basics of cardiac MDCT: techniques and contrast application. *Eur Radiol*, 2005, 15(Suppl 2), B2–B9.

16. Daniell, A.L., et al. Concordance of coronary artery calcium estimates between MDCT and electron beam tomography. *Am J Roentgenol*, 2005, 185, 1542–5.

17. Agatston, A.S., et al. Quantification of coronary artery calcium using ultrafast computed tomography. *J Am Coll Cardiol*, 1990, 15, 827–32.

18. Schroeder, S., et al. Reliability of differentiating human coronary plaque morphology using contrast-enhanced multislice spiral computed tomography: a comparison with histology. *J Comput Assist Tomogr*, 2004, 28, 449–54.

19. Kopp, A.F., et al. Reproducibility and accuracy of coronary calcium measurements with multidetector row versus electron-beam CT. *Radiology*, 2002, 225, 113–9.

20. Greenland, P., S.C. Smith, Jr., and S.M. Grundy. Improving coronary heart disease risk assessment in asymptomatic people: role of traditional risk factors and noninvasive cardiovascular tests. *Circulation*, 2001, 104, 1863–7.

21. Rumberger, J.A., et al. Electron beam computed tomographic coronary calcium scanning: a review and guidelines for use in asymptomatic persons. *Mayo Clin Proc*, 1999, 74, 243–52.

22. Grundy, S.M. Coronary plaque as a replacement for age as a risk factor in global risk assessment. *Am J Cardiol*, 2001, 88(Suppl), 8E–11E.

23. Arad, Y., et al. Prediction of coronary events with electron beam computed tomography. *J Am Coll Cardiol*, 2000, 361253–60.

24. Arad, Y., et al. Predictive value of electron beam computed tomography of the coronary arteries. 19-month follow-up of 1173 asymptomatic subjects. *Circulation*, 1996, 93, 1951–3.

25. Greenland, P., and J. Stamler. Comparison of low risk and higher risk profiles in middle age to frequency and quantity of coronary artery calcium years later. *Am J Cardiol*, 2004, 94, 367–9.

26. Smith, Jr., S.C., P. Greenland, and S.M. Grundy. AHA Conference Proceedings. Prevention Conference V: Beyond secondary prevention: identifying the high-risk patient for primary prevention: executive summary. American Heart Association. *Circulation*, 2000, 101, 111–6.

27. P. Greenland, et al. Coronary artery calcium score combined with Framingham score for risk prediction in asymptomatic individuals. *JAMA*, 2004, 291, 210–15.

28. Raggi, P., and D.S. Berman. Computed tomography coronary calcium screening and myocardial perfusion imaging. *J Nucl Cardiol*, 2005, 12, 96–103.

29. Raggi, P., et al. Progression of coronary calcium on serial electron beam tomographic scanning is greater in patients with future myocardial infarction. *Am J Cardiol*, 2003, 92, 827–9.

30. Achenbach, S., et al. Influence of lipid-lowering therapy on the progression of coronary artery calcification: a prospective evaluation. *Circulation*, 2002, 106, 1077–82.

31. Hecht, H.S., and S.M. Harman. Evaluation by electron beam tomography of changes in calcified coronary plaque in treated and untreated asymptomatic patients and relation to serum lipid levels, *Am J Cardiol*, 2003, 91, 1131–4.

32. Screening for Heart Attack Prevention and Education (SHAPE) Task Force report in www.VP.org or www.AEHA.org.

33. Shaw, L., P. Raggi, and T.Q. Callister. Establishing cost effective thresholds for coronary disease screening: a predictive model with risk factors and coronary calcium. *Prog Cardiovasc Dis*, 2003, 46, 171–84.

34. Georgiu, D., et al. Screening paients with chest pain in the emergency department using electron beam computed tomography: a follow-up study. *J Am Coll Cardiol*, 2001, 38, 105–10.

35. Third Report on the National Cholesterol Education Program (NCEP) Expert Panel on Detection, Evaluation, and Treatment of High Blood Cholesterol in Adults (Adult Treatment Panel III) final report. *Circulation*, 2002, 106, 3143–421.

Coronary Artery Stenoses: Detection, Quantitation and Characterization

4

4.1 Introduction

Multidetector computed tomography (MDCT) is a potentially useful tool for a comprehensive study of the complex aspects of coronary artery lesions. It allows, on one hand, the obtention of a noninvasive coronary angiography, or a "luminogram" of the arteries, where the degree of obstruction of lesions can be assessed. On the other hand, MDCT is not limited to this analysis but it is also able to give information on the arterial wall itself and on the extent and components of atherosclerotic plaques (Figure 4.1).

When compared with conventional angiography, noninvasive coronary angiography by MDCT has shown a fairly high degree of accuracy for the detection of significantly obstructive coronary artery lesions in both native vessels[1–4] (Table 4.1) and arterial or venous grafts[5–11]. Reliability of MDCT studies has increased from the introduction of 4-slice systems, the first allowing an adequate visualization of coronary arteries[12–17], to those with 16[18–24] and, more recently, 64 detectors[1–4].

Nevertheless, noninvasive coronary angiography by MDCT still has limitations[25], particularly in the presence of heavily calcified lesions, metallic implants in the coronary tree, or in patients with irregular heart rhythm. These have been mentioned as causes of the somewhat reduced diagnostic accuracy of MDCT when compared with invasive angiography as a reference method. Cases of discrepancy, however, should not be entirely attributed to MDCT, but limitations of conventional angiography must also be considered[26–33]. Predictive positive value of MDCT for the presence of significantly obstructive coronary artery lesions is around 80% in most comparative studies[4,18–22], which can be considered as suboptimal. Invasive angiography, on its part, has also shown discrepancies in the assessment of coronary lesions when compared with the more accurate method of intravascular ultrasound (IVUS), which evidences a number of lesions missed by angiography[27–29,34,35]. The mentioned predictive positive value of MDCT should thus be tested against IVUS, provided the possibility of actual false negatives of coronary angiography (Figures 4.2 and 4.3).

MDCT can even be considered superior to invasive angiography in some aspects[2] as is allows the obtention of unlimited views, in contrast with angiography. In fact, MDCT does

RUBÉN LETA-PETRACCA
SANDRA PUJADAS
GUILLEM PONS-LLADÓ

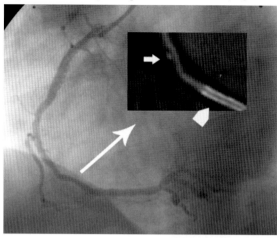

FIGURE 4.1 Conventional angiography of the right coronary artery showing mild luminal narrowing in the distal segment suggesting the presence of a lesion. The MDCT image corresponding to this segment (inset) also demonstrates luminal narrowing, but more importantly, it also shows the atherosclerotic plaque (arrow) and it allows us to assess its composition. A coronary stent is also seen distally (arrowhead), which passes undetected at the conventional angiography.

Table 4.1 Accuracy of MSCT-64 to detect coronary stenosis >50% in comparison to QCA. Adapted from Leber, et al.[2]

Segments	Sensitivity	Specificity
Proximal–mid segments	75%	97%
Distal segments	67%	97%
All segments	73%	97 %
Lesions requiring revascularization	83%	–
+++ Calcified segments	75%	89%
0/+ Calcified segments	72%	98%

not render "projections" but "sections" of the coronary artery tree with any angulation and, most important, in a retrospective way, after the whole cardiac volume has been acquired. Images obtained from MDCT may include, thus, cross-sectional views of the vessels (Figure 4.4) which are not available in angiographic studies, this allowing a more detailed analysis of the magnitude of lesions[36], similarly to IVUS, with which MDCT has shown good correlation in the first comparative studies performed to date[2,37–40].

4.2 Analyisis of Coronary Artery Lesions

The assessment of coronary artery lesions by MDCT implies different, important aspects of their relevance, as is the magnitude of obstruction, and the composition of atherosclerotic plaques and its morphological features, all related with the stability of lesions.

A systematic analysis of a coronary artery MDCT study must take[41] into consideration the following steps:

1. Analyisis of images reconstructed from different phases of the cardiac cycle, in order to choose those where the coronary arterial tree is best filled with contrast and where movement artifacts are the least (Figure 4.5) (see also Chapter 1).

2. A complete review of axial images that constitute the cardiac volume, paying attention to cardiac anatomy, degree of opacification of chamber and walls of the heart (Figure 4.6), and aspect of extracardiac structures[42] (Figure 4.7).

3. Optimization of images aimed to improve the visualization of coronary arteries by using specific postprocessing protocols and by the appropriate setting of window width/level controls (Figure 4.8).

4. Analysis of the coronary artery tree, for which the following systematization is fundamental:

   a. Exam of the anatomical distribution of coronary arteries, aimed to identify normal variants (Figure 4.9) and congenital abnormalities of the origin of vessels (see also Chapter 2).

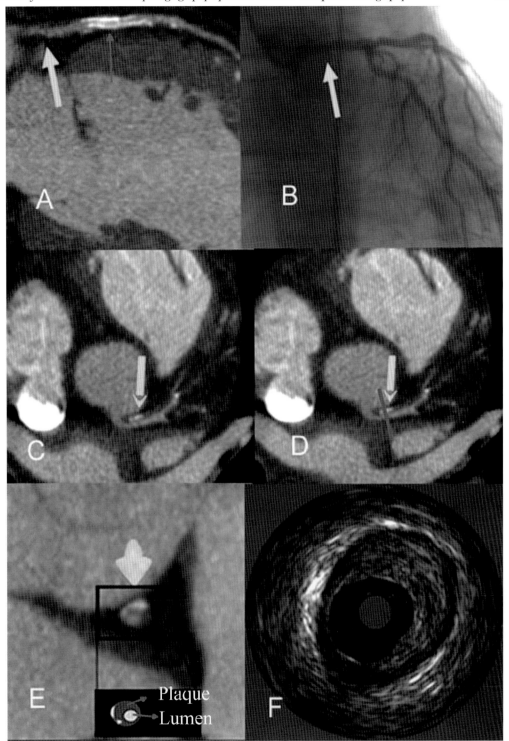

FIGURE 4.2 Left main coronary artery lesion in a patient with a previous stent placed in the left anterior descending artery. Curved multiplanar reconstruction (MPR). (A) shows the left main coronary artery with a mild stenosis (large arrow) and also a stent in the proximal left anterior descending artery (small arrow). MPR image is concordant with the invasive coronary angiogram (B). However, axial images (C) suggest a more severe lesion than showed by the conventional angiogram. A transverse section of the left main artery (E) obtained from an axial plane (D) allows not only a more precise assessment of the severity of the stenosis, but also an insight of the components of the plaque. This particular view of a lesion (E) cannot be obtained by means of a conventional angiogram and can only be achieved using IVUS (F), which finally confirms the MDCT estimation in this particular patient.

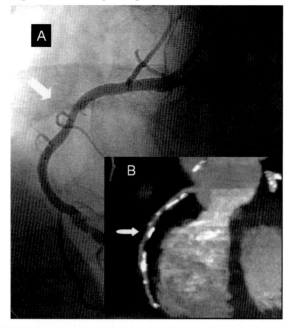

FIGURE 4.3

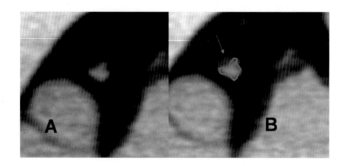

FIGURE 4.4

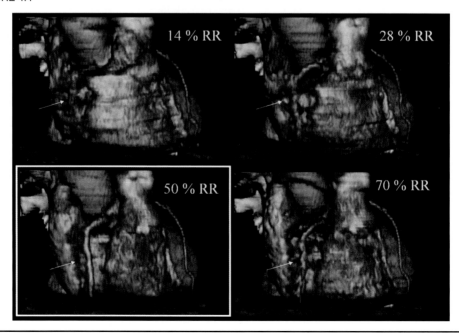

FIGURE 4.5

F. 4.3. A: Invasive coronary angiogram showing the proximal and middle segments of the right coronary artery with no evidence of obstruction. B: MDCT angiography of the same segments of the vessel. Although MDCT image may be more limited in the evaluation of the luminogram of the vessel due to coronary artery calcifications, it provides a better assessment of the extent and severity of coronary atherosclerotic disease. Note the presence of calcified coronary plaques (arrow in B) that are otherwise missed by invasive coronary angiography.

F. 4.4. Transverse section of the left anterior descending artery (A) showing an eccentric noncalcified atheromatous plaque (arrow), that can be clearly distinguished from the lumen area (line) (B).

F. 4.5. Cardiac volume from a study reconstructed from different phases of the cardiac cycle. Note that the right coronary artery is best depicted in the images obtained at 50% of the R-R cycle (left lower panel), the other phases showing severe motion artifacts.

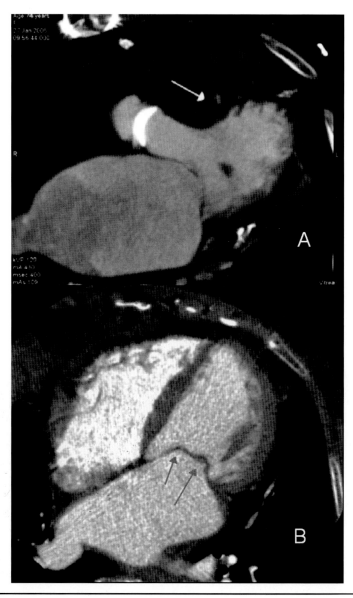

FIGURE 4.6 A: An optimally contrasted MDCT study showing a high degree of opacification of the left cardiac chambers as opposed to the right ones, in which no contrast is visualized, these allowing a good assessment of the septal branch course (arrow). B: Analysis of axial images allows detection of cardiac conditions other than coronary artery disease such as this rheumatic mitral stenosis found by chance in a patient with chest pain. Note the doming shape of the anterior leaflet in diastole (arrows).

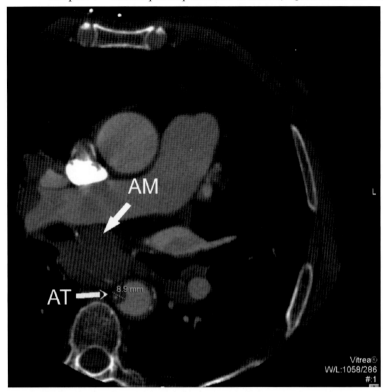

FIGURE 4.7 Routine analysis of axial images before the assessment of coronary arteries allows the detection of potential coexistent abnormalities with clinical relevance. In this image an adenopathic mass (AM) was found in a patient with an unsuspected malignant lung neoplasia. This patient also showed a severe aortic atherosclerosis with a protruding atheromatous plaque (AT) in the descending aorta.

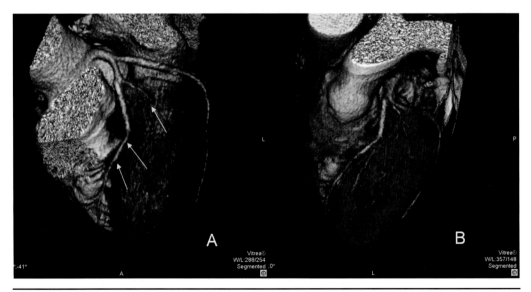

FIGURE 4.8 Optimization of imaging parameters is mandatory in order to perform an appropriate analysis of coronary arteries lesions by MDCT. Figure (A) shows how an inappropriate adjustment of the window W/L leads to an inaccurate visualization of the diagonal branches of the left anterior descending artery (arrows). Figure (B) shows the same image with an optimized adjustment, which allows the evaluation of these arteries.

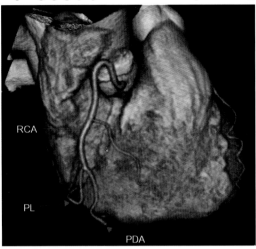

FIGURE 4.9 Normal variant of the right coronary artery (RCA) easily detected on the 3D volume rendering, which shows the artery bifurcating at the acute cardiac margin–proximally to the *crux cordis*—into a posterolateral branch (PL) and a posterior descending artery (PDA).

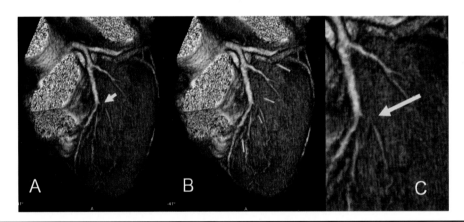

FIGURE 4.10 A: Apparent stenosis of the second diagonal branch of the left anterior descending artery (arrow). B: Knowledge of the coronary anatomy (arterial and venous) and an accurate analysis of the image (C) help to identify the course of the great cardiac vein crossing over the proximal segment of this diagonal branch (arrow), leading to the false appearance of arterial stenosis in this 3D volume rendering image.

   b. Detection and localization of coronary artery lesions, carefully avoiding sections and angulations or interposed structures with potential image artifacts (Figure 4.10).

   c. Evaluation of composition and morphology of the lesion.

   d. Qualitative and quantitative assessment of obstruction of the vessel caused by the lesion.

A classification of atherosclerotic coronary artery lesions is possible by applying this systematic analysis of MDCT. This classification can be made according to the following aspects:

- The vessel involved: native artery, arterial or venous bypass graft, stented arterial segment.
- The location: proximal, middle or distal portions of the vessel. According to the topography of the lesion, more descriptive terms can be used: ostial (Figure 4.11), at a bifurcation (Figure 4.12), at an anastomosis (Figure 4.13); and, in the case of stented vessels: in-segment (proximal or distal to the stent) (Figure 4.14) or in-stent (into the stent itself).
- The extension of the lesion: focal or diffuse (Figures 4.15 and 4.16), eccentrical or concentrical (Figures 4.17 and 4.18).

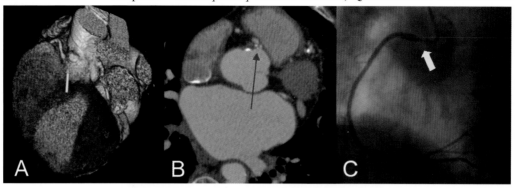

FIGURE 4.11 Right coronary ostial lesion. A: 3D Volume rendering reconstruction shows an important decrease in lumen size and density, suggesting the presence of a lesion (arrow). B: Axial image showing the severity of the ostial lesion (arrow) as well as its mixed composition (calcific/fibrous lesion). C: Invasive coronary artery angiogram confirms a severe right coronary ostial stenosis (arrow).

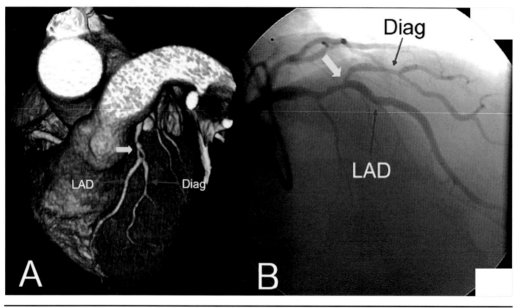

FIGURE 4.12 Bifurcational lesion involving the middle segment of the left anterior descending artery and a diagonal branch. A: 3D volume rendering reconstruction showing not only lumen narrowing but also a positive remodeling lesion and its mixed composition: hypondense areas reflecting lipid or fibrous components and a hyperdense area due to focal calcification (yellow arrow). B: Conventional coronary angiogram confirming the lesion. LAD: left anterior descending artery; Diag: diagonal artery.

- The degree of obstruction[43]:

  1. Nonsignificant stenoses (less than 50% of the vessel lumen, including mild and moderate degrees of obstruction) (Figures 4.19 and 4.20).
  2. Borderline stenoses (50–70%) (Figure 4.21).
  3. Significant stenoses (more than 70%, including critical—subocclusive—and occlusive lesions (Figures 4.22–4.24).

- The components of the lesion[37,39,43–45]:

  1. Thrombotic lesions (Figure 4.25).
  2. Noncalcified, mixed, or "soft" lesions: adipose (Figure 4.26) and fibroadipose (Figure 4.27).
  3. Calcified lesions: fibrocalcified (Figures 4.27 and 4.28) and calcified (Figures 4.27 and 4.29). The calcium component of the lesion can be focal, diffuse, eccentrical or concentrical.

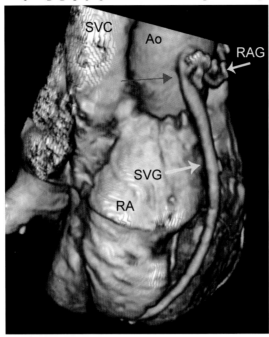

FIGURE 4.13 3D volume rendering reconstruction of a patient with a composite coronary artery bypass graft. A saphenous vein graft (SVG) to the right coronary artery is seen with its proximal anastomosis on the aortic root (Ao). A radial artery graft (RAG) is also seen anastomosed to the proximal segment of the venous graft. In the venous graft—distal to this vein-to-artery anastomosis—a narrowing lumen is observed (red arrow). RA: right atrium; SVC: superior vein cava.

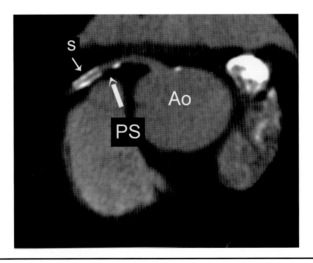

FIGURE 4.14 Oblique MPR reconstruction showing a coronary stent (S) and an in-segment lesion (arrow) adjacent to its proximal edge. PS: pre-stent. Ao: aorta.

A particular case is that of non-atherosclerotic coronary artery lesions, including both congenital and acquired abnormalities of these vessels, as abnormal origin (see also Chapter 2), fistulae, intramyocardial bridges, or coronary aneurysms.

4.2.1 Diagnostic tools of MDCT applied in the study of coronary artery lesions

4.2.1.1 Axial images

Images resulting from the axial acquisition of MDCT are the basis on which multiplanar

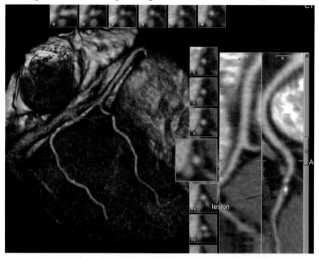

FIGURE 4.15

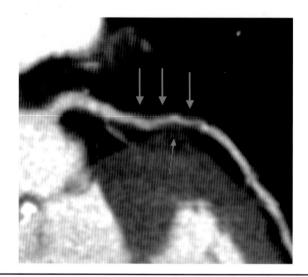

FIGURE 4.16

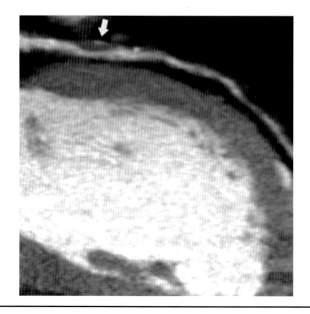

FIGURE 4.17

F. 4.15.   Curved MPR reconstruction. Focal coronary lesion (arrow) in the proximal segment of the posterolateral branch of the right coronary artery, showing a mixed composition of the plaque.

F. 4.16.   Curved MPR reconstruction. Coronary artery lesion involving an extense proximal segment of the left anterior descending artery (arrows). Notice that the plaque shows an exclusively fibrolipid composition.

F. 4.17.   Curved MPR reconstruction showing a focal, eccentric, coronary lesion in the proximal left anterior descending artery. Although mainly fibrolipidic, a core probably composed by calcium is also seen (arrow).

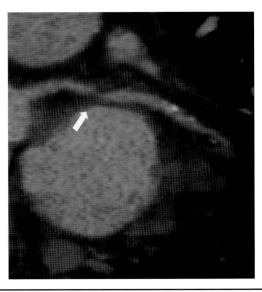

FIGURE 4.18 Curved MPR reconstruction showing a focal, concentric, noncalcified coronary lesion in the circumflex artery (arrow).

reconstructions can be performed[41,46]. Axial images contain all the information from the body of acquired data, and are devoid of any loss of information or the presence of artifacts that eventually degrade reconstructed images. Although limited to a two-dimensional view, axial images constitute an adequate method for the analysis of cardiac and thoracic anatomy (Figure 4.7) and, due to its excellent resolution, also for the evaluation of the components of coronary atherosclerotic lesions (Figure 4.30). A systematic review of axial images is advisable as it permits the evaluation of the quality of the study in terms of contrast opacification and the detection of potential artifacts leading to interferences on the reconstructed images.

4.2.1.2 3D volume render reconstruction

The diagnosis of severity of a coronary artery stenosis by MDCT is based, as in the case of invasive angiography, on a qualitative estimation of the lesion. This evaluation starts, in MDCT, with the exam of the 3D volume render reconstruction[41,47], as it allows a quick visualization of the distribution of the coronary

arterial tree, where it is easy to identify the presence of normal variants (Figure 4.9), abnormal origin, and course of the vessels (Figure 4.31) or intramyocardial bridges (Figure 4.32).

This 3D reconstruction gives a "vascular image," which basically consists of the amount of contrast filling the lumen of the vessel. Thus, the presence of a noncalcified atherosclerotic lesion, characterized by a reduction in the luminal density (Figure 4.33), is promptly detected, although 3D images are not the preferred method for the estimation of the severity of the lesion. The localization of lesions in particular segments of the vessels (Figures 4.34 and 4.35) is easily done with 3D reconstruction, as is its extension, the involvement of branches (Figure 4.36), and the detection of potentially confusing structures such as coronary veins, (Figure 4.10), paraortic lymph nodes, or aortic wall atherosclerotic plaques (Figures 4.37 and 4.38).

3D reconstruction is very helpful in cases of occlusive lesions, where the lack of filling of the distal vessel (Figure 4.24), or its filling through alternative collateral circulation (Figure 4.39),

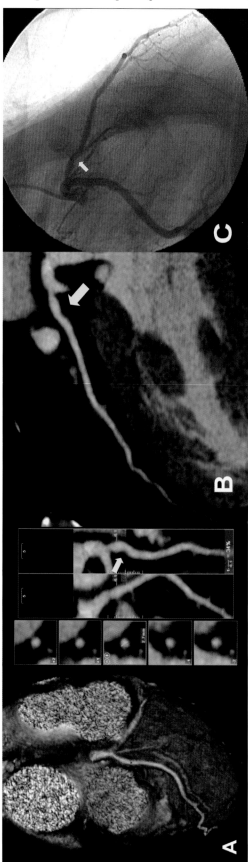

FIGURE 4.19 Mild coronary lesion in the proximal segment of the left anterior descending artery. A: 3D volume rendering reconstructions and curved MPR, showing a fibrofatty plaque (arrow). B: Curved MPR reconstruction of the left anterior descending artery showing the exact localization of the coronary lesion. C: Conventional coronary angiogram in the right anterior oblique projection confirming the findings of the MDCT.

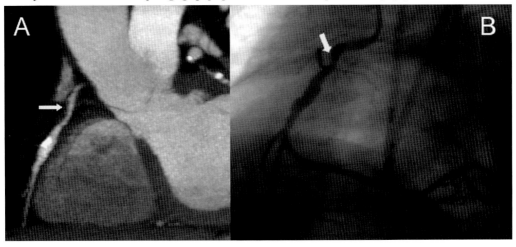

FIGURE 4.20 Eccentric, noncalcified, moderate coronary lesion in the proximal segment of the right coronary artery (arrow). A: Maximum intensity projection (MIP) image. B: Invasive coronary angiogram.

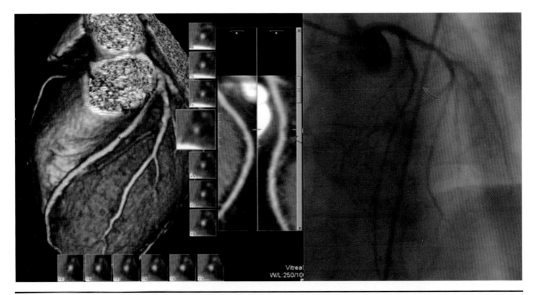

FIGURE 4.21 Coronary lesion of borderline significance in the middle segment of the left anterior descending artery (arrow). A: 3D volume rendering and curved MPR reconstructions. B: Invasive coronary angiogram.

which in some cases can be imaged in itself (Figure 4.40), is easily detected.

The detection of calcium in atherosclerotic plaques is also easily made with 3D images (Figure 4.41), although its presence, particularly when concentric in appearance, considerably limits the usefulness of this technique for the analysis of the magnitude of obstruction to flow caused by the lesion (Figure 4.42). Finally, other highly dense structures which may lie adjacent to coronary arteries, such as metallic clips (Figure 4.43), pacemaker leads, or valve

prostheses (Figure 4.44), are also recognized on 3D reconstructions.

4.2.1.3 Multiplanar reconstruction (MPR)

Coronary artery lesions are eccentrical in relation to the vessel lumen[48,49]. Conventional coronary angiography obviates this fact by means of performing a (limited) number of different projections[33]. The approach by MDCT consists of obtaining sections of the vessels on multiple orientations by means of MPR techniques, not limited to the axial plane.

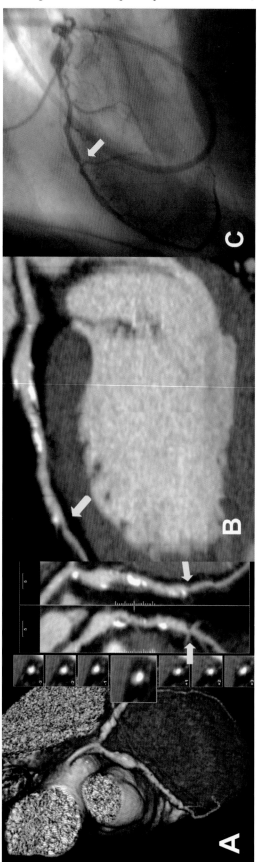

FIGURE 4.22 Coronary lesion resulting in a significant stenosis in the distal segment of the left anterior descending artery. A: 3D volume rendering and curved MPR reconstructions. B: Curved MPR reconstruction of the left anterior descending artery. Note that besides this significant lesion (arrow) there is also an extensive atherosclerosis of the rest of the vessel with focal calcifications, which are not so well distinguished by the conventional coronary angiogram (C).

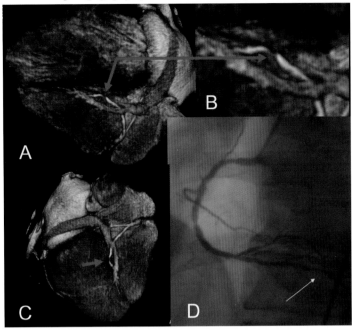

FIGURE 4.23 Subocclusive lesion in the distal segment of the posterior descending artery (arrow). A and C: 3D volume rendering reconstructions. B: Detailed 3D image of the lesion. D: Conventional coronary angiogram showing the same lesion (arrow).

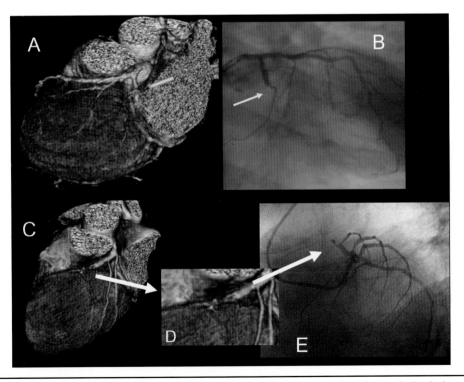

FIGURE 4.24 Occlusive coronary lesions. A: 3D volume rendering reconstruction of an occlusive lesion of the proximal segment of the circumflex artery (arrow). B: Corresponding conventional coronary angiogram in the anteroposterior projection. C: 3D volume rendering reconstruction of an occlusion of the middle segment of the left anterior descending artery. D: Detailed image of the lesion. E: Corresponding conventional coronary angiogram in a left anterior oblique "spider" view.

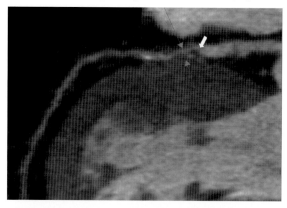

FIGURE 4.25

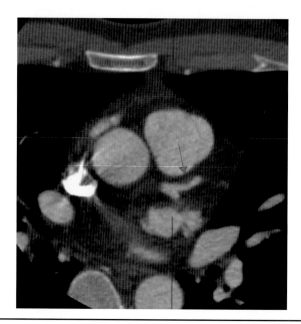

FIGURE 4.26

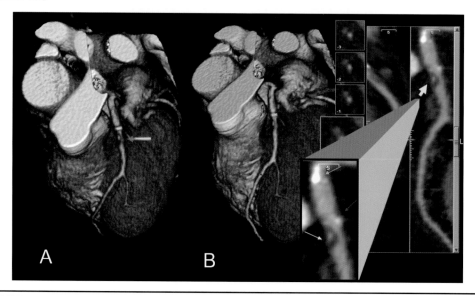

FIGURE 4.27

F. 4.25. Curved MPR reconstruction showing a significant lesion of the middle segment of the left anterior descending artery (thin symmetrical arrows) with irregular borders and a component with a very low value of Hounsfield units, probably corresponding to thrombus (thick arrow). The study was obtained from an old lady presenting with an acute coronary syndrome who rejected an invasive coronary angiogram.

F. 4.26. Lipid-rich lesion of the proximal segment of the left anterior descending artery (arrow) on an axial image.

F. 4.27. Coronary lesion in the middle segment of the left anterior descending artery. A: 3D volume rendering reconstruction. B: 3D volume rendering and curved MPR reconstruction in which the lesion is clearly seen (thick yellow arrow). MPR detailed reconstruction (inset) shows the mixed composition (fibrolipid) of the principal lesion (thin yellow arrow) but other minor lesions also are observed: fibrocalcific (red arrow) and calcific plaques (blue arrow).

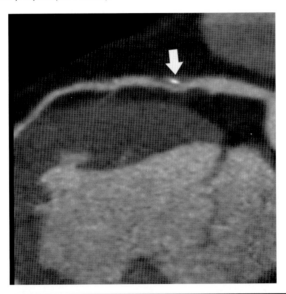

FIGURE 4.28 Curved MPR reconstruction showing a fibrocalcific lesion in the midsegment of the left anterior descending artery (arrow).

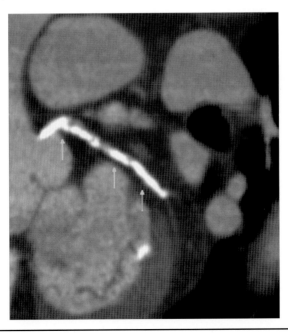

FIGURE 4.29 Curved MPR reconstruction showing diffuse coronary atherosclerosis with calcified lesions (arrows) involving the proximal and middle segment of the circumflex artery.

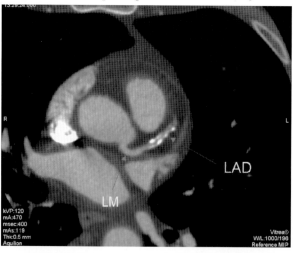

FIGURE 4.30

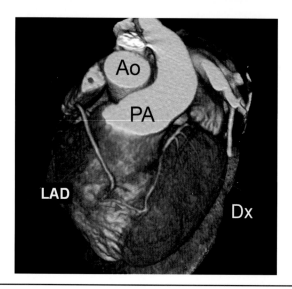

FIGURE 4.31

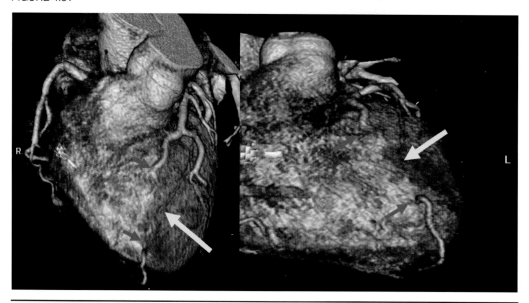

FIGURE 4.32

F. 4.30. Axial image allowing a rapid analysis of atherosclerotic plaque composition. In this image an extensive—highly calcified—lesion of the left anterior descending artery is shown (LAD). LM: left main artery.

F. 4.31. Congenital anomalous origin of the left anterior descending (LAD) artery from the right coronary artery. The LAD artery arises from the right coronary artery and courses anteriorly to the right ventricular outflow tract, finally reaching its normal course along the anterior interventricular groove. Diagonal branches (Dx) arise from this distal portion. Ao: ascending aorta; PA: pulmonary artery.

F. 4.32. 3D volume rendering reconstructions showing a myocardial bridge over the middle segment of the left anterior descending artery (yellow arrows). Observe the proximal and distal ends of the tunneled arterial segment (red arrows).

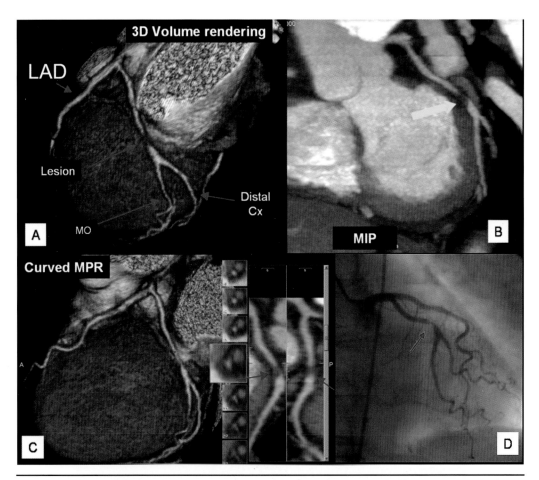

FIGURE 4.33 Noncalcified lesion in the midsegment of the circumflex artery. A: 3D volume rendering image showing an abrupt fall in density at the middle segment of the circumflex artery indicating the presence of a noncalcified lesion. Assessment of the lesion severity may be performed on MIP (B) and curved MPR (C) images. Conventional coronary angiogram confirms MDCT findings (D). Cx: circumflex artery; LAD: left anterior descending artery; MO: marginal oblique artery.

By means of different modalities of MPR, a clear view of both the lumen and the wall of the vessel is possible, this facilitating a detailed analysis of lesions.

There are two modalities of MPR: oblique and curved[47]. In the *oblique* mode, a view of the vessel is obtained by angulating the study plane with any orientation over the axial plane, guided by the course of the vessel on the latter (Figure 4.45). MPR on a *curved* format can be obtained manually by signaling the center of the vessel through consecutive axial images. By computing this information, the system provides a two-dimensional image of the course of the vessel independent of the anatomic distribution of the artery (Figure 4.46). As this method is time-consuming and the final image is largely dependent on an appropriate centering

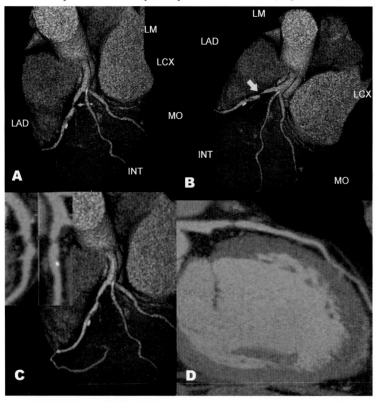

FIGURE 4.34

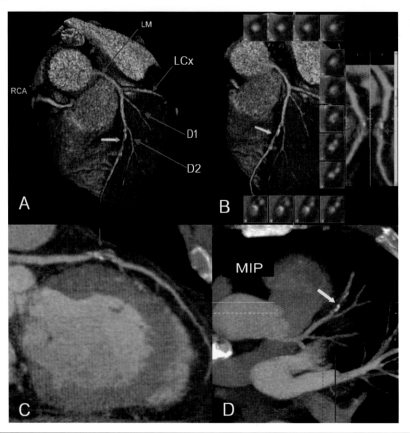

FIGURE 4.35

F. 4.34. Noncalcified lesion in the left anterior descending artery (LAD). A and B: 3D volume rendering reconstructions in which a proximal decrease in luminal density is observed (yellow arrow). C: Automatic curved MPR obtained by selecting the left anterior descending artery in the 3D image (green line). Noncalcified lesion in the proximal segment is shown in 2 orthogonal sections of the vessel (arrows). D: Automatic curved MPR reconstruction of the left anterior descending artery, allowing a clear identification of the lesion in the proximal segment of the vessel (arrows). INT: intermediate artery; LAD: left anterior descending artery; LCx: left circumflex artery; LM: left main; MO: marginal obtuse artery.

F. 4.35. Lesion in the mid-distal segment of the left anterior descending artery. A: 3D volume rendering reconstruction shows—immediately distal to the second diagonal branch (D2)—a narrowing of the vessel and a reduction of the luminal density, indicating the presence of a lesion (yellow arrow). B: By manually selecting the left anterior descending artery in the 3D image (green line), a curved automatic MPR of such artery is obtained; the orthogonal projections of the vessel show the lesion severity (red arrows) and its mixed composition (fibrolipidic plaque with focal calcification). C: Automatic curved MPR reconstruction of the left anterior descending artery allows a clear identification of the lesion in the middle segment of the vessel (arrows). D: MIP images showing the severity of the lesion (arrow) and the lack of involvement of the origin of the second diagonal branch, which arises immediately proximal to the lesion.

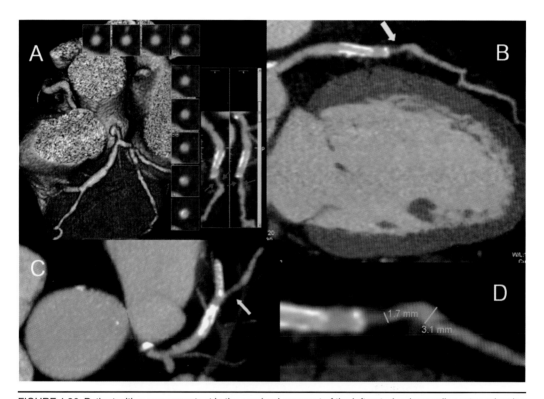

FIGURE 4.36 Patient with a coronary stent in the proximal segment of the left anterior descending artery showing a lesion at the origin of the first diagonal branch. A: 3D volume rendering and curved MPR in which the lesion is observed (arrows). B: Curved MPR reconstruction of the diagonal branch clearly shows a proximal lesion. C: MIP images do not suggest a significant lesion. D: Detailed curved MPR image in which the lesion stenosis is quantified (45%; distal reference vessel diameter: 3.1 mm; minimum luminal diameter: 1.7 mm).

of the markers by the operator[47], alternative automatic curved MPR modalities have been developed. In these modes, the operator puts a single electronic mark on any segment of a particular vessel on a 3D volume image. This gives the system the signal for a tracking of the entire course of the vessel, based on the distinctive value of Hounsfield units due to the contrast present in the artery (Figure 4.47).

MPR techniques allow the assessment of important aspects of coronary lesions, such as their extension along the vessel, cross-sectional appearance, and composition (Figure 4.27). Also, images obtained by MPR permit the

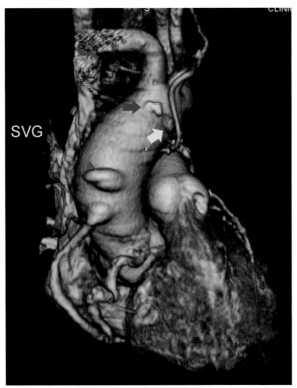

FIGURE 4.37

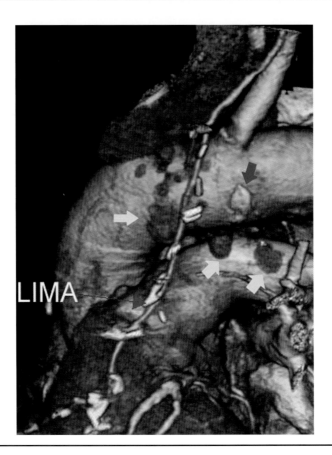

FIGURE 4.38

F. 4.37. 3D volume rendering reconstruction showing the stump from an occluded aortocoronary venous graft (red arrow), as well as two different potentially confusing images: paraaortic node (yellow arrow) and calcified atheromatous plaque (blue arrow). SVG: saphenous vein graft.

F. 4.38. 3D volume rendering reconstruction of a patient with a left internal mammary artery graft. Paraaortic images as a paraaortic node (yellow arrows) and calcified atheromatous plaque (blue arrow) are seen, which is important to recognise in a systematic study.

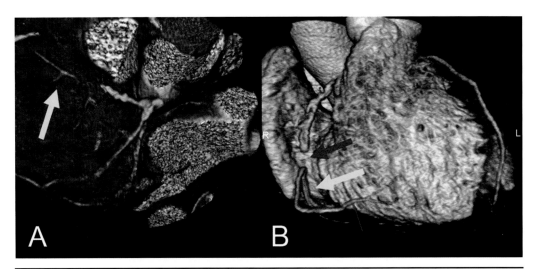

FIGURE 4.39 Vessel filling distally to a coronary artery occlusion. A: 3D volume rendering reconstruction showing a proximal occlusion of the left anterior descending artery (blue arrow). Partial vessel filling distal to the occlusion is observed (yellow arrow). B: 3D volume rendering reconstruction from another patient showing an occlusion of the middle segment of the right coronary artery (blue arrow). Note that in this case—as opposed to the previous one—there is a complete distal vessel filling after the arterial occlusion (yellow arrow) that even involves the marginal acute branch (red arrow).

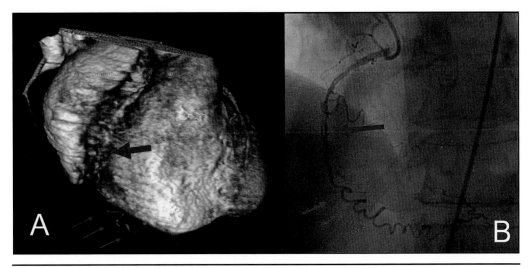

FIGURE 4.40 A: 3D volume rendering reconstruction showing an occlusion of the middle segment of the right coronary artery (blue arrow). Note that the right coronary artery provides collateral circulation to its distal segment (red arrows). B: Conventional invasive coronary angiogram.

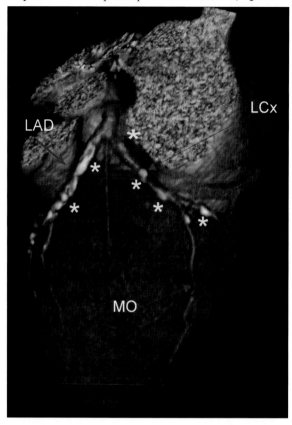

FIGURE 4.41 Multivessel diffuse atherosclerotic coronary artery disease. 3D volume rendering reconstruction showing numerous calcified plaques (yellow asterisks). LAD: left anterior descending artery; LCx: left circumflex artery; MO: marginal obtuse branch.

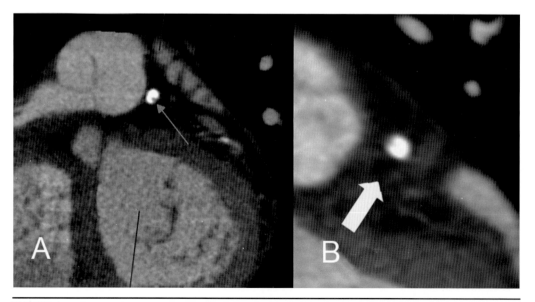

FIGURE 4.42 Concentric coronary artery calcification. A: Transversal section of the middle segment of the left anterior descending artery, where a partial volume artifact due to calcification allows only a small segment of the artery wall to be seen (arrow). B: Calcification involving the whole arterial wall in a different patient. Although in both cases the stenosis seems to be significant, it is impossible to accurately establish the severity of the obstruction.

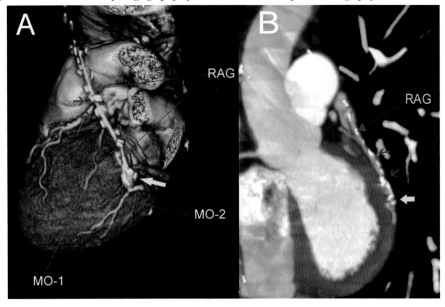

FIGURE 4.43 Metallic clips of a radial artery coronary graft with distal anastomosis to the second marginal obtuse branch of the circumflex artery. A: 3D volume rendering reconstruction showing marked metallic clips artifacts around the coronary graft (blue arrows). As shown in the MIP image (B), at the distal anastomosis the artifact is very pronounced (yellow arrow), hampering a correct evaluation of the presence of lesions at this site. MO: marginal obtuse artery; RAG: radial artery graft.

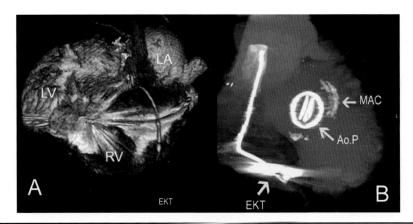

FIGURE 4.44 A: 3D volume rendering reconstruction showing the striking artifact produced by a pacemaker lead (EKT) placed into the right ventricle. B: Potential sources of artifacts in MDCT: pacemaker lead (EKT), mechanical aortic prosthesis (Ao.P), mitral annulus calcification (MAC). LA: left atrium; LV: left ventricle; RV: right ventricle.

measurement of the obstruction caused by an atherosclerotic lesion, as true cross-sectional views of the stenotic site can be obtained (Figure 4.47), similarly to invasive IVUS techniques.

4.2.1.4 Maximal intensity projection (MIP) and volume rendering techniques

Both of these are based on computed spatial summation of a series of consecutive slices (slab) presented as a two-dimensional image. MIP and volume rendering techniques can be applied to axial or MPR images (Figure 4.48)[41,46,47]. In MIP images those structures with high X-ray attenuation are highlighted, while the rest are lessened. In volume render techniques, the intensity of pixels in the image is the result of applying different algorithms of opacification of structures depending on the relative position of their voxels and their density.

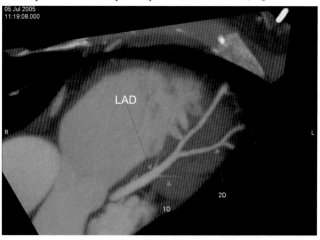

FIGURE 4.45 Oblique MPR showing the left anterior descending artery (LAD) and the diagonal branches (1D and 2D).

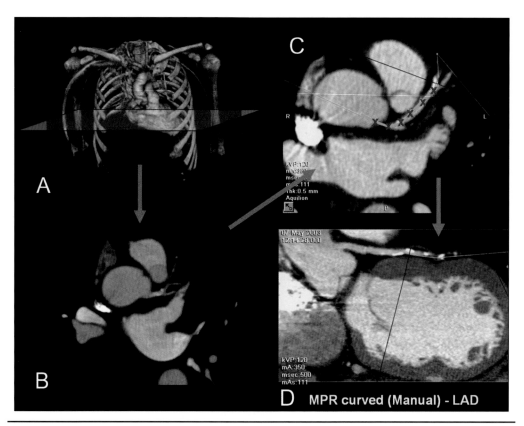

FIGURE 4.46 Curved MPR obtained manually. Using the axial images (A and B), a tracking of the vessel through different axial planes is performed by means of "seeds" (C), resulting in an image that unfolds the whole artery (D). Although this image does not correspond to a true anatomical plane, it is very useful for the assessment of the vessel from a single image.

Both modalities are useful in the analyisis of coronary lesions, particularly MIP images, as their appearance is similar to those of invasive coronary angiography (Figure 4.33b).   MIP are helpful in the study of the right coronary artery (RCA), when images are interfered with banding artifacts (Figure 4.49) in those lesions located at bifurcational sites, as the origins of

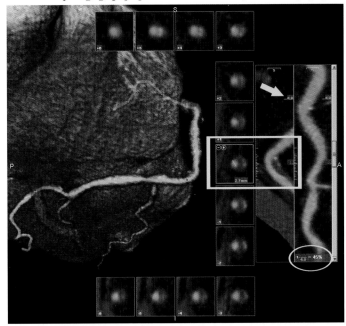

FIGURE 4.47 Quantification of a coronary lesion in a curved MPR reconstruction. Vessel diameter is assessed by means of a transverse section at the proximal reference segment of the vessel (yellow arrow) and at the lesion site (yellow open square), obtaining a stenosis percentage (45% in this case).

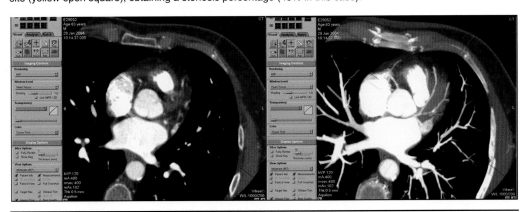

FIGURE 4.48 MIP projection. Left panel shows an MPR oblique view of a thin section (1 mm) depicting the aortic root. When an MIP projection is applied, performing a spatial summation of consecutive sections (16 mm), the left anterior descending artery, the first diagonal branch and the proximal right coronary artery are all also included in the same image.

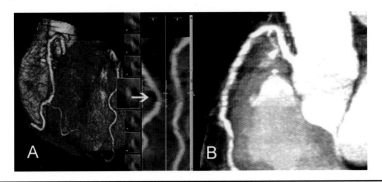

FIGURE 4.49 Right coronary artery. A: Curved MPR reconstruction of a case with banding artifacts interfering with the assessment of the vessel lumen in the middle segment (arrow). MIP image (B) provides improved visualization of the artery.

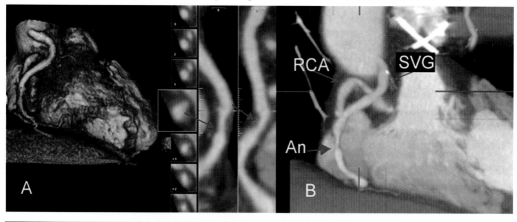

FIGURE 4.50 Distal anastomotic lesion of a saphenous aortocoronary graft. The lesion can be visualized in the curved MPR reconstruction (A), although its exact location at the distal anastomosis of the graft (An) is more clearly defined on the MIP image (B). RCA: right coronary artery; SVG: saphenous vein graft.

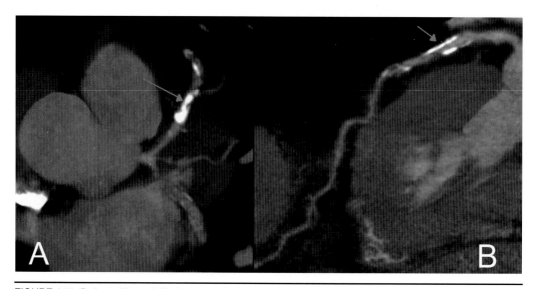

FIGURE 4.51 Patient with a calcified coronary lesion. MIP images (A) highlight structures with high density which overshadow those less dense, this impeding to accurately assess the severity of the lesion. On the other hand, curved MPR (B) clearly shows that the lesion, in this case, is not significant.

diagonal and marginal branches, and—together with curved MPR—in the analysis of bypass grafts (Figure 4.50).

MIP images also have limitations, particularly when structures causing great X-ray attenuation, such as calcium or metal, are present in the wall of the arteries. These materials are highlighted by MIP techniques, and the estimation of the actual magnitude of lesions from the image is interfered, even when the thickness of the slab from which the MIP is formed is reduced to a minimum (Figure 4.51).

4.2.2 Reading a MDCT coronary angiography

MDCT has a high spatial resolution—submillimetric—which, together with the aid of robust tools for the analysis of images such as 3D volume rendering or MPR, makes the technique highly reliable in the study of coronary arteries[3,4].

The detection of coronary artery lesions from a technically adequate MDCT study is not particularly troublesome, in contrast with their quantification, which is a more complex process. Although coronary artery lesions are frequently detected on a first inspection of axial images or 3D reconstructions, the reader must always be sure that there are no artifacts present that interfere with the image of the vessel.

There are different sources of artifacts in a MDCT coronary angiography which are frequently responsible for those instances of disagreement between this technique and conventional invasive angiography[25,41].

4.2.2.1 Imaging artifacts

4.2.2.1.1 Artifacts dependent on the optimization of images (windowing artifacts)

The detection of coronary lesions from a MDCT study frequently starts by inspecting the 3D volume render reconstructed images, where the anatomical course of coronary arteries can be identified, and potential interference with other structures, such as the coronary veins, can be detected. Important in this sense is, in addition to using the appropiate visualization protocol, to set the adequate window width/level of the image, and the systematic exam of the axial—non reconstructed—images to prevent false diagnosis (Figure 4.10).

4.2.2.1.2 Movement artifacts Movement artifacts do appear when images have been retrieved from an inadequate phase of the cardiac cycle (Figure 4.5), as in ventricular systole, ventricular diastole (when extremely short due to increased heart rate), or atrial contraction period. Increased heart rate, even when regular, can induce these artifacts by the shortening of systolic and diastolic periods and also by the increased translational movements of the heart. Premature atrial or ventricular beats, or arrhythmias in general, may also be causes of these artifacts.

Movement artifacts show as blurred images leading to a poorly defined outline of segments of the vessels, particularly the RCA and left circumflex (LCx) arteries, due to their anatomic relationship with the atria and their course along different anatomic planes.

As discussed on Chapter 1, the use of beta-blocking agents, oxygen or sedatives may prevent the appearance of movement artifacts. Once the study is acquired, a careful exam of the heart rhythm, suppressing those eventual irregular beats, and the selection of the most adequate cardiac phases for reconstruction are essential for avoiding movement artifacts.

4.2.2.1.3 Reconstruction or banding artifacts These artifacts do appear when the heart rate changes significantly during the acquisition time of the exam. The dispersion of the cardiac cycle duration may lead to an image reconstruction composed of slices corresponding to slightly different phases of the cardiac cycle, this resulting in images with an indented outline of the cardiac structures in a stepped shape (Figure 4.52). Banding artifacts are prone to appear at the end of the acquisition time, when the regularity of the cardiac cycle frequently tends to dissipate. For this reason, the middle and distal segment of the coronary arteries are the locations most often affected by these artifacts.

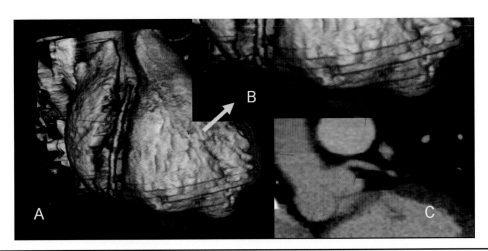

FIGURE 4.52 Reconstruction artifact. A and B: 3D volume rendering reconstructions with the typical stepped image involving those slices acquired at the late stage of the study. C: Pseudostenosis due to a reconstruction artifact.

Again, a careful analysis after the acquisition allows for the identification of those cardiac cycles with the most variable length regarding the basal one, which can be excluded from the reconstruction of images. In those cases where images are still suboptimal after this editing process, volume render or MIP techniques may allow for a partial analysis of segments of the coronary arteries, presenting with these banding artifacts (Figure 4.49).

4.2.2.1.4 Partial volume artifacts Partial volume artifacts are caused by the presence of structures with high X-ray attenuation coefficient located in proximity to the vessels. They are visualized as high density ("bright") images causing a blooming effect that overshadows surrounding structures, this frequently leading to a magnification of lesions.

Partial volume artifacts are characteristic of calcified coronary artery lesions (Figure 4.42). In cases where calcification involves all the circumference of the vessel and grows concentrically, the signal from the true vascular lumen may be completely obscured by the artifact, but in eccentrically calcified lesions there may be also interference, this limiting the diagnostic accuracy of MDCT in the assessment of severity of coronary artery lesions.

Partial volume artifacts may be minimized by means of different tools, such as curved MPR or MIP with reduced slab thickness (Figure 4.51).

4.2.2.1.5 Streak artifacts These artifacts are induced by large metallic or highly dense structures, such as valve prostheses, pacemaker leads or accumulation of iodinated contrast,

and are visualized as bright, linear star-shaped structures (Figures 4.44 and 4.53–4.54).

Streak artifacts can be the cause of apparently obstructive coronary lesions in the proximal segments of the coronary arteries, in the presence of aortic valve prostheses or accumulation of contrast at the superior vena cava, or also, in distal segments of the left anterior descending (LAD) artery in patients with pacemaker leads placed in the apical region of the right ventricle.

4.2.2.1.6 Artifacts dependent from the body type Signal-to-noise ratio is usually reduced in obese patients, this limiting the quality of images[3]. In addition, these individuals frequently present with larger heart chambers, where the contrast dilutes and, as a result, opacification of the coronary tree is decreased. In these cases, local hypodense segments of the distal coronary arteries are frequently seen that can be taken as diffuse coronary lesions (Figure 4.55).

A careful selection of both the contrast volume and the radiation parameters can diminish the presence of these artifacts and improve image quality.

4.2.2.1.7 Artifacts dependent from respiratory movements The performance of an adequate breath-hold by the patient is still an essential aspect in MDCT coronary angiography, even after the introduction of the recent 64-slice systems. When either a pathological state or the lack of cooperation from the patient leads to an incorrect breath-hold maneuver, respiratory artifacts are introduced in the image in the form of linear blurred signals distorting the

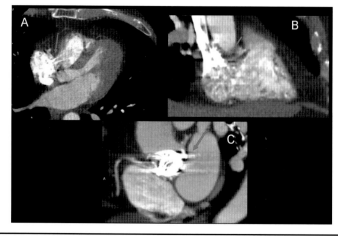

FIGURE 4.53 Lineal artifacts. A and B: persistence of high contrast concentration in the inferior vena cava due to an inappropriate wash out (arrows). C: Aortic metallic prosthesis.

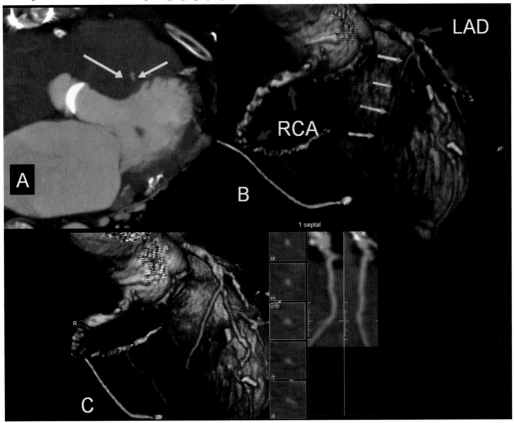

FIGURE 4.54 Optimal contrast opacification of the cavities during the acquistion of a non-invasive coronary study. A: Axial image. Appropriate contrast wash out results in the absence of contrast opacification in the right cardiac chambers, allowing to more accurately delineate the course of the first anterior septal branch through the interventricular septum (yellow arrows). B: 3D volume rendering reconstruction allows to clearly visualize the first anterior septal branch, as well as the right coronary artery (RCA) course. C: With these optimized images different analysis tools, such as automatic curved MPR, might also be easily used.

outline of structures. Respiratory artifacts can be distinguished from reconstruction artifacts by the fuzzy appearance of the lung parenchyma (Figure 4.56).

4.2.2.2 Assessment of the magnitude of coronary artery lesions

A comprehensive study of a coronary lesion by any method implies, in practice, the assessment of the degree of obstruction which can be determined qualitatively and quantitatively.

In invasive coronary angiography, a coronary stenosis is estimated by comparing the size of the coronary lumen in the involved segment with that of a proximal segment of the same vessel, at a level presumably free of lesions. The reduction of the vascular lumen expressed in percentage defines the degree of stenosis. Experimental studies[50] based on coronary flow reserve measurements have established that a 50

to 70% stenosis can be considered as significant.

Although, in practice, this estimation has been traditionally performed qualitatively, a quantitative analysis can be applied by means of the so-called Quantitative Coronary Angiography (QCA) method (Figure 4.57). This type of analysis, however, has some limitations[32,51–55] (Figure 4.58). On one hand, QCA measurements are performed on a two-dimensional image obtained from an angiographic projection corresponding, in fact, to three-dimensional structures. On the other hand, atherosclerosis is, by nature, a diffuse process[33], and obstructive lesions are frequently eccentrical in distribution[48].

These limitations have lead to the development of analysis based on intravascular diagnosing methods: intravascular ultrasound (IVUS)[34] and Doppler and pressure probes. These tools have shown to considerably improve the ability

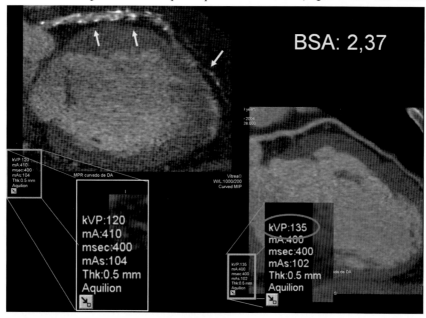

FIGURE 4.55 Noninvasive coronary studies of 2 obese patients with comparable body surface area. Left: signal-to-noise ratio is not appropriate due to an incorrect radiation adjustment of the study. Right: patient in whom the radiation given was correctly adjusted, resulting in good quality image for the analysis. BSA: body surface area.

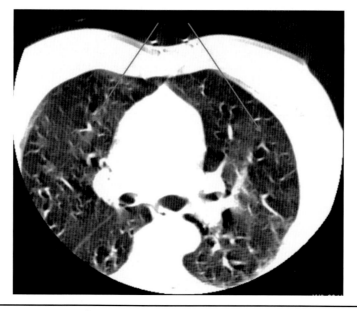

FIGURE 4.56 Fuzzy appearance of the lung fields (arrows) in a case with inadequate breath-hold during the acquisition.

to quantify coronary stenoses[34,35]. In addition to being invasive and expensive, however, these methods are faced with one main limitation, as is their dependency from angiography: IVUS and Doppler probes are usually applied only in those cases where there is angiographic suspicion of the presence of a lesion. As it is known, the angiographic "luminogram" may actually miss the presence of a lesion[26–33,52,55], a case in which a further investigation by these methods would not be performed (Figures 4.57 and 4.58).

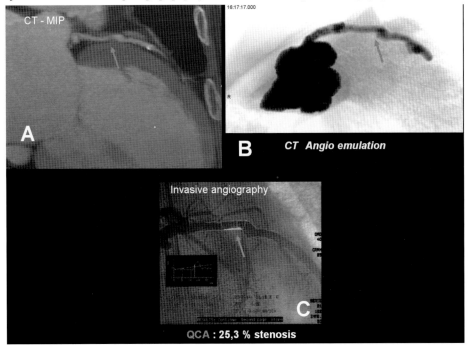

FIGURE 4.57 Atherosclerotic lesion in the middle segment of the left anterior descending artery. MIP image (A) shows a nonsignificant lesion (arrow), which is confirmed in the angio-emulation view (B), obtained by means of postprocessing analysis, as well as at an invasive quantitative coronary angiography (QCA) (C).

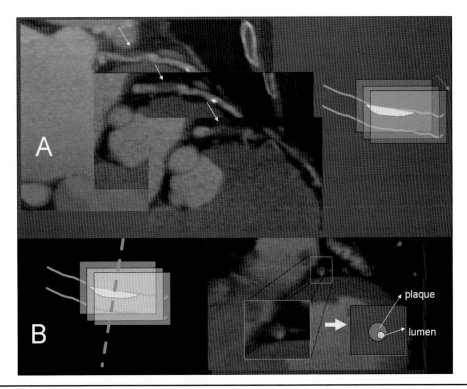

FIGURE 4.58 A: Fine slices parallel to the center of the vessel on its longitudinal axis showing an apparently higher degree of the obstruction than that observed on the simple MIP image (background frame in the series). B: Cross-sectional submillimetric slice (dashed line) at the level of the lesion demonstrating its eccentricity and actual obstructive character, in contrast with the rather benign QCA estimation (see Figure 4.57).

For all of these reasons, MDCT coronary angiography is considered to have a potential role in the study of coronary artery disease[36], provided that it does not have some of the incoveniences discussed previously. Some of these distinctive features are the following:

1. The analyisis of the percentage of vessel stenosis can be performed on true sections of the artery, this obviating the limitations of projections (Figure 4.46 and 4.47).
2. MDCT allows precise definition of the boundaries between healthy and diseased vessel segments, which derives a more accurate measurement of the true coronary stenosis. This represents an advantage over invasive angiography, which is limited in the case of diffuse coronary atherosclerosis[28,33] (Figure 4.16).
3. The MDCT analysis allows for the obtention of multiple views of the vessels on multiple orientations, many of them not affordable by invasive angiography, which is advantageous in the case of eccentrical lesions. In this sense, MDCT can be considered as the first noninvasive technique able to obtain images of the coronary arteries similar to those from IVUS (Figures 4.4, 4.47, 4.58, 4.59). This permits the measurement of luminal area and burden plaque of a coronary segment (Figure 4.59), and the evaluation of the process of remodeling of the diseased vessel (Figure 4.60). These parameters have proven to correlate adequately with invasive measurements[2,40,56,57].
4. In contrast to IVUS, MDCT analysis of cross-sectional views of the vessels can easily be applied to all segments of the coronary artery tree, and as an off-line study, this

does not imply additional acquisitions and irradiation (Figure 4.2).

Despite these advantages, MDCT also has some limitations, particularly on the purely angiographic aspects of the exam, that have not been definitively overcome by the continuous technological advances. The more relevant of these limitations are as follows:

1. The reliability of MDCT depends on the type of vessel (native artery, stented vessel, venous or arterial graft) and the diameter of the segment to be studied.
2. Dependency from the regularity of heart rate, the adequacy of the breath-hold, and the presence of high X-ray attenuation structures into or near the vessel wall, such as calcification, metallic clips, or stents[25]. These limitations have resulted in 10 to 15% of unreadable vessel segments in different studies[3,20,22].
3. Relatively high potential for interobserver variability, due to several causes: largely different equipment facilities at present between centers (4,8,16 and 64 detectors) (Figure 4.61), different capacities between systems with apparently similar technological features, and limited training of most observers at present, provided the recent introduction of the technique.

4.2.2.2.1 Assessment of native coronary arteries
Diagnostic accuracy of MDCT for the detection and assessment of lesions on native coronary arteries is high in proximal and middle segments of the vessels[1,2] (Figure 4.62), while it is somewhat less when studying distal segments or secondary branches[20], provided their reduced diameter and contrast opacification. The left main (LM) (Figures 4.2

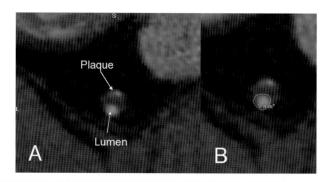

FIGURE 4.59 A: Cross-sectional view of a coronary artery with an eccentric atherosclerotic lesion. B: Minimal luminal area calculation.

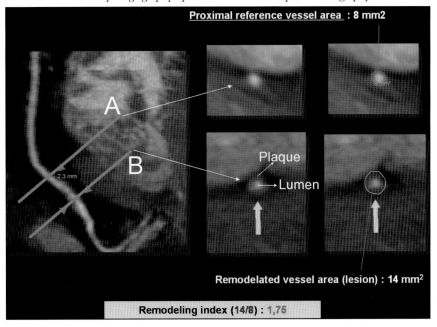

FIGURE 4.60 Remodeling index calculation. Curved MPR reconstruction (left panel) showing a normal coronary segment (A) and a diseased segment (B) with an enlargement of the vessel diameter. Cross-sections of these sites are seen on the middle panels, and measurements of the vessel areas on the right panels. Note that this is a lesion with a highly atheromatous concentric plaque lesion with positive remodeling of the vessel (index: 1.75).

and 4.63) and LAD arteries (Figure 4.17) in particular, are the most readily visualized ones and, therefore, they exhibit a low rate of non-evaluable segments in different studies[1,2,20,21]. The RCA and LCx coronary arteries, and all secondary branches (Figure 4.64), present with smaller diameters than the previous ones, and they course through a larger amount of axial MDCT planes (Figure 4.5) than the LM and LAD, this resulting in a higher frequency of reconstruction and movement artifacts. For these reasons, the accuracy of MDCT in RCA and LCx is somewhat lower than in the case of LM and LAD[1,2,20,21].

In the absence of severe calcification of the arterial wall, coronary artery lesions can be detected and quantified by MDCT (Figure 4.47). However, there can be some difficulty in distiguishing critical subocclusive lesions from occlusive ones[20] with filling of the distal vessel through collateral circulation (Figures 4.39B and 4.65). This is due to limitations in the visualization of tiny collateral vessels and to the lack of dynamic information of MDCT that prevents assessment of the mode of filling of a particular vessel segment.

In despite of this, MDCT can provide useful anatomical information in cases of occlusive lesions[58], when percutaneous intervention is considered. In this sense, MDCT allows a more accurate measurement of the length of the occlusion[58] (Figure 4.66) than that from invasive angiography, a parameter closely related with success of the procedure. Also, the shape of the proximal site of the occlusion (tapered or wedged), the degree of calcification of the lesion, the presence of perivascular circulation (bridges), and the existence of branching vessels arising from the occlusion are all data potentially obtainable by MDCT that can be highly useful in planning therapeutic strategies[58].

4.2.2.2.2 Assessment of coronary artery bypass grafts

Coronary artery bypass grafts (CABG) are more amenable to MDCT imaging, due to their larger diameter and lower pulsatile movements along the cardiac cycle, than native arteries (Figure 4.67). Reports on diagnostic accuracy of MDCT in CABG have shown values of sensitivity and specificity over 95% for the presence of lesions in these vessels[5–11,59].

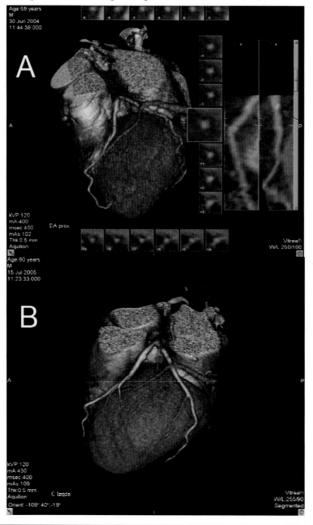

FIGURE 4.61 Noninvasive coronary angiography studies from the same patient, performed with a 16-slice (A) and a 64-slice (B) unit. Note the improved image quality in study B which can be attributed to the more advanced 64-slice system. While both studies were performed at similar heart rates and equivalent radiation doses, breath-hold time in study B was much shorter than in A (from 28 to 10 seconds), and contrast volume given was lower (from 130 to 70 cc).

The technique provides, in particular, adequate information on the course of the vessel graft, the distal anastomosis (Figures 4.68–4.71), and the native vascular bed from both the grafted and non-grafted arteries (Figures 4.72 and 4.73). MDCT allows a reliable detection of different CABG obstructive lesions (Figures 4.74–4.80). A relevant aspect of MDCT study of CABG is its ability to readily define the status of patency or occlusion of the graft (Figures 4.81–4.83), being in this sense even superior to invasive angiography[11], that not exceptionally leads to a false diagnosis of graft occlusion when it has not been selectively catheterized.

Occluded aortocoronary venous grafts present with patent proximal stump at the aortic wall that gives a characteristical image at MDCT (Figure 4.81). Although not filled with contrast, the segment of the vessel distal to the occlusion site can also be visualized as a low-density fibrous tract (Figure 4.82).

Arterial grafts pose some limitations to MDCT study, as is the presence of metallic clips in mammary artery and, particularly, in radial artery grafts[60], that interfere with the visualization of lesions. Also, the non-dynamic

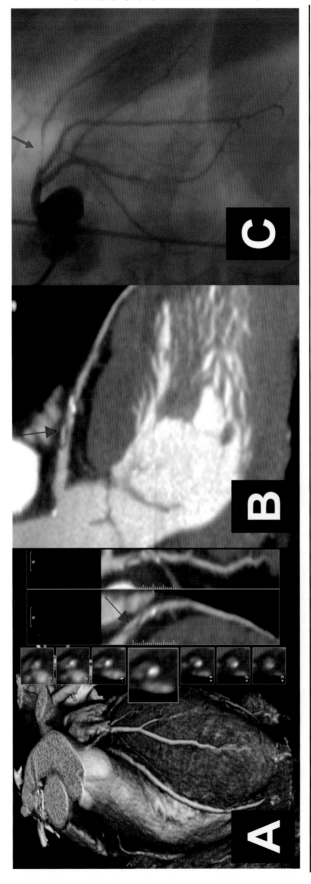

FIGURE 4.62 Coronary lesion with significant stenosis ($>70\%$) at the proximal segment of the intermediate artery. A: 3D volume rendering and curved MPR images with two orthogonal views of the lesion (arrow). B: Curved MPR showing the lesion (arrow) with an orientation similar to the one of the invasive angiography (C), which shows an otherwise comparable degree of obstruction.

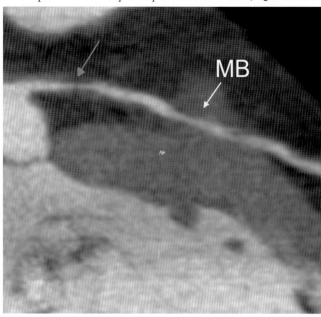

FIGURE 4.63 Extensive fibrolipid lesion of the left main artery (dark arrow) with a myocardial bridge (bright arrow, MB) at the proximal segment of the left anterior descending artery.

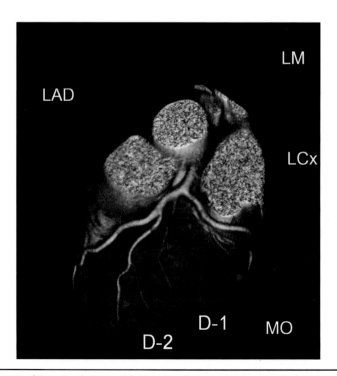

FIGURE 4.64 Influence of the vessel diameter in the visualization of coronary arteries. Large branches, as the left main (LM), left anterior descending (LAD), and left circumflex (LCx) arteries present with a higher degree of contrast opacification than the smaller ones, such as the diagonal (D-1) and marginal obtuse (MO) branches. Observe the improved opacification of the second diagonal branch (D-2) in respect to the D-1, indicating that the former has a larger vessel diameter.

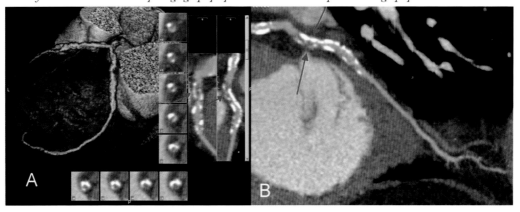

FIGURE 4.65 A: 3D volume rendering and curved MPR of the circumflex and marginal obtuse arteries. A lesion with high calcium contents and irregular borders is seen. Observe the marked reduction of vessel luminal density inside the lesion (red arrows) suggesting occlusion of the vessel at this site, as was subsequently proven at invasive angiography. B: The extended view of the vessel in this curved MPR shows adequate contrast opacification of a large extension distally to the lesion, a usual finding by MDCT when, despite a proximal occlusion, such a vessel segment is supplied by collateral circulation (see also Figure 4.39). In the present case, the short extension of the occlusion, together with the visualization of the distal vessel, could falsely lead to the diagnosis of subocclusive lesion; the absence of any contrast opacification inside the lesion highly favors the diagnosis of vessel occlusion.

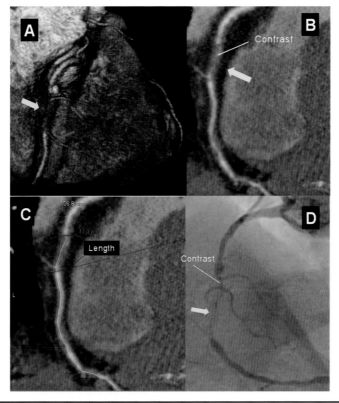

FIGURE 4.66 Occlusive lesion at the middle segment of the right coronary artery. A: 3D volume rendering showing an abrupt fall of vascular density at the site of the occlusion (yellow arrow). Two acute marginal branches can be visualized emerging from this occluded segment (blue arrows). Also, a small calcification in the proximal end of the occlusion (red arrow) is detected. B: Curved MPR that shows partial recanalization of the occlusion with evidence of some contrast media present in the vascular lumen. C: The length of the occlusion is easily assessed with appropriate tools in the curved MPR images. D: Image corresponding to the invasive coronary angiography confirming the mentioned findings: partial recanalization of the occluded segment and presence of two branches (blue arrows) emerging from the site of the involved segment. Angiography is, however, limited in the detection of calcification and in the measurement of the length of the occlusion due to the projection of the vessel.

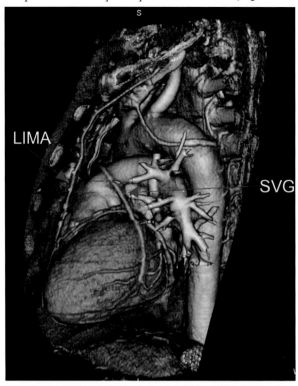

FIGURE 4.67 Clear, wide field-of-view of thoracic structures on a 3D volume rendering by MDCT provides excellent anatomical information on the situation and course of coronary arterial or venous grafts. LIMA: left internal mammary artery; SVG: saphenous vein graft.

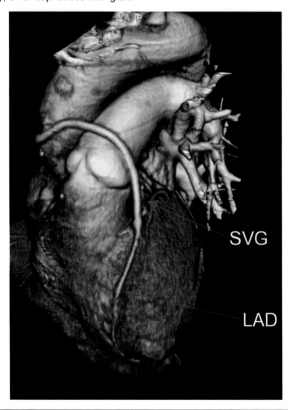

FIGURE 4.68 3D volume rendering reconstruction of a saphenous vein graft (SVG) anastomosed to the left anterior descending artery (LAD).

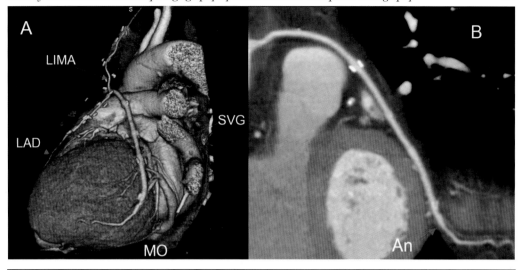

FIGURE 4.69 A: 3D volume rendering reconstruction of a saphenous vein graft (SVG) anastomosed to the marginal obtuse artery (MO). B: Curved MPR reconstruction shows absence of obstructive lesions in the graft.

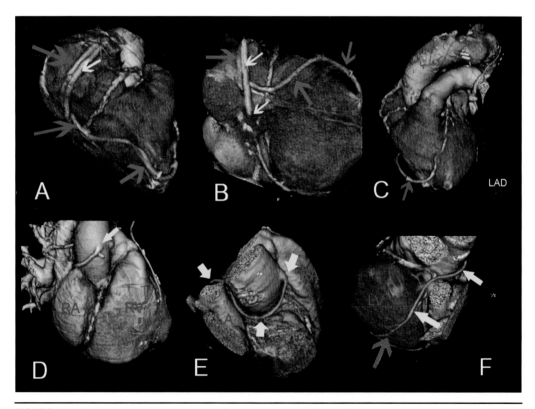

FIGURE 4.70 Unusual anatomical courses of aortocoronary grafts. A–C: Images from a patient showing two saphenous vein coronary grafts, one of them to the posterior descending artery (yellow arrows) and the other (red arrows) to the left anterior descending artery (LAD), following an unusual course through the inferior wall of the heart. D–F: Images from a different patient showing a saphenous vein aortocoronary graft (yellow arrows) to the marginal obtuse artery (red arrow) with a retroaortic course. LA: left atrium; LV: left ventricle; RA: right atrium; RV: right ventricle.

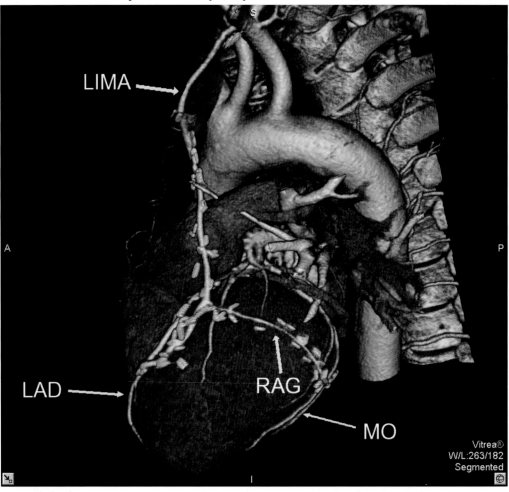

FIGURE 4.71 Left internal mammary artery coronary graft (LIMA) with anastomosis to the left anterior descending artery (LAD). The proximal end of a radial artery graft (RAG) is anastomosed to the LIMA graft and distally to the marginal obtuse artery (MO).

nature of MDCT makes difficult the assessment of competitive flow (Figure 4.84) or vasospasm in the arterial graft.

4.2.2.2.3 Assessment of stented coronary arteries
MDCT may provide useful information on different aspects of stented arteries. It allows a fast and accurate assessment of the patency[61] of the stented segment by evaluating the presence (or not) of contrast filling in distal portions of the vessel (Figures 4.85 and 4.86). Also, in-segment lesions located at the proximal and distal borders of the stent can be assessed (Figures 4.87–4.90).

As metallic structures, coronary artery stents present with a high X-ray attenuation co-efficient causing partial volume effects that degrade the image quality of the vessel lumen[62] (Figure 4.86). Thus, the exam is limited in the

evaluation of in-stent stenoses[63,64], particularly in those devices with small diameter values[61]. The composition of the stent has somewhat less influence on MDCT images[64]. It has been reported that, in contrast with native vessels, up to 23% of coronary artery stented segments are not evaluable by MDCT[61]. Limitations in the assessment of stented vessels appear when the diameter of the stent is smaller than 3 mm, or the strut is thicker than 140 μm. This leads to a suboptimal diagnostic accuracy for the detection of in-stent lesions, even when using advanced MDCT technology[64].

On the other hand, in the case of devices with large diameter (>4–5 mm), a MDCT study may allow the visualization of the process of in-stent neointimal hyperplasia (Figures 4.89, 4.91 and 4.92), which opens the way for a future

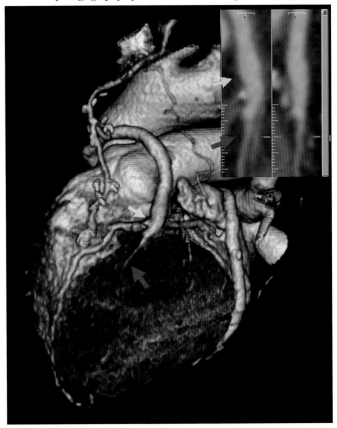

FIGURE 4.72 3D volume rendering and curved MPR reconstructions of a saphenous vein graft to a diagonal branch. Note the small diameter of the native distal vessel, which is markedly disproportionate when compared to the graft.

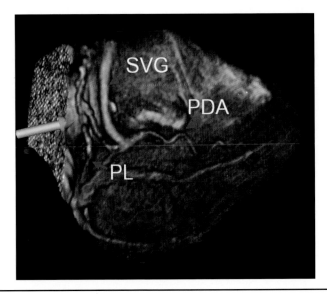

FIGURE 4.73 Significant *de novo* obstructive lesion (yellow arrow) in the posterolateral branch (PL) in a patient previously treated by means of a venous coronary graft (SVG) to the posterior descending artery (PDA).

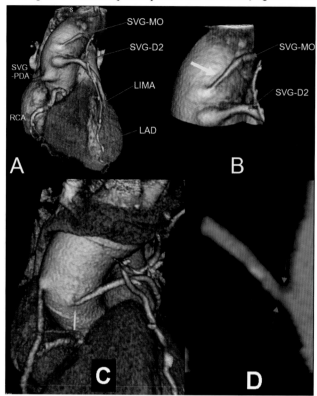

FIGURE 4.74 A and B: Images from a patient with a quadruple coronary bypass showing an obstructive lesion in the proximal anastomosis of the venous graft to the marginal obtuse branch (SVG-MO) (yellow arrow, in B). Compare the diameter of this segment of the vessel to the one of the saphenous vein graft to the second diagonal branch (SVG-D2). C and D: Images from a different patient with a stenotic lesion of a saphenous vein aortocoronary graft, visualized on both the 3D volume rendering (yellow arrow, in C) and the curved MPR reconstruction (red arrows, in D). LAD: left anterior descending; LIMA: left internal mammary artery; RCA: right coronary artery; SVG-PDA: saphenous vein graft to the posterior descending artery.

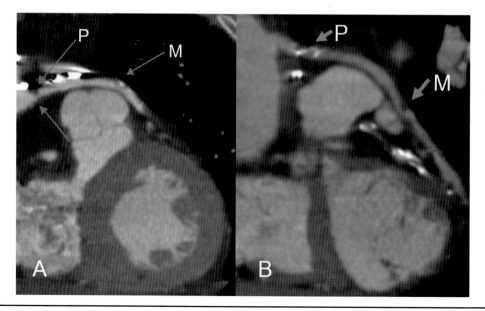

FIGURE 4.75 Significant stenotic lesions of saphenous vein grafts in two different patients. A: Noncalcified proximal lesion (P) and a fibrocalcified lesion in the middle segment (M). B: Calcified proximal lesion (P) and a fibrolipid lesion in the middle segment (M).

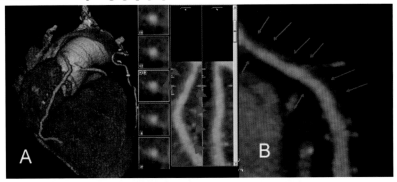

FIGURE 4.76 A: 3D volume rendering and curved MPR reconstruction showing a diffuse lesion of a saphenous vein graft to the posterior descending artery. B: Detail of the involved segment.

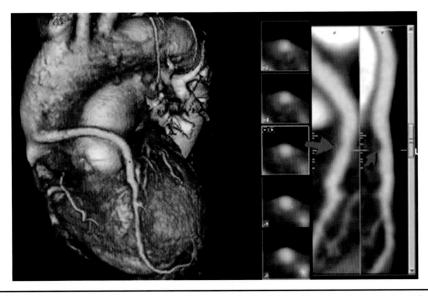

FIGURE 4.77 3D volume rendering and curved MPR reconstructions showing a saphenous vein graft to the left anterior descending artery with a nonsignificant lesion in its distal segment (red arrows).

potential application of the technique, as does the follow-up of stents in large vessel segments such as the left main coronary trunk[65].

4.2.2.3 MDCT study of the components of coronary artery atherosclerotic plaques

In addition to the detection and quantification of coronary artery lesions, MDCT also permits an adequate visualization of the vessel wall[36–38], this allowing the study of morphological features of atherosclerotic plaques and the distinction between their components. This can be done due to the different behavior of organic tissues in terms of attenuation of X-ray, expressed by Hounsfield units[39,43,44].

Studies on cadaveric hearts[44] have established the ranges of Hounsfield units that define different types of coronary atherosclerotic lesions:

- Predominantly adipose atherosclerotic plaques: ≤60 HU
- Mixed plaques: 61–119 HU
  - Fibroadipose: 61–90 HU
  - Fibrocalcified: 91–119 HU
- Predominantly calcified atherosclerotic plaques: ≥120 HU

This information on plaque composition is potentially relevant, provided the histological features known to distinguish high-risk atherosclerotic plaques, such as their large lipidic core, thin fibrous cap, and presence of inflammatory phenomena[66–68]. Importantly, these lesions do not necessarily present with significant obstruction to flow, but with eccentrical

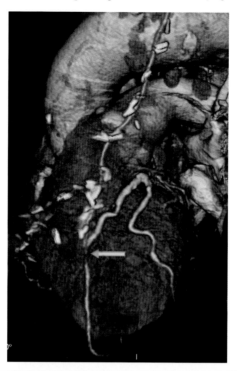

FIGURE 4.78

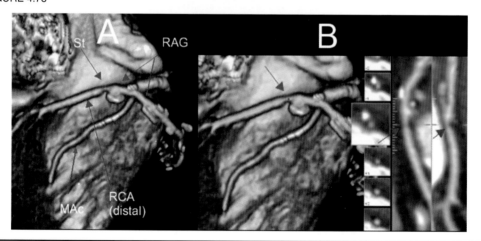

FIGURE 4.79

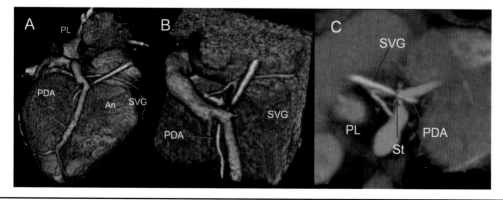

FIGURE 4.80

F. 4.78.   3D volume rendering reconstruction of a mammary artery graft showing a significant stenotic lesion at the site of the anastomosis of the graft (yellow arrow).

F. 4.79.   A: 3D volume rendering reconstruction showing a significant stenotic lesion (St) at the distal anastomosis of a radial artery graft (RAG) to the right coronary artery (RCA). B: Curved MPR reconstruction confirming the stenosis previously visualized in the 3D reconstruction (red arrows). MAc: marginal acute branch of the right coronary artery.

F. 4.80.   Images from a patient with a significant stenotic lesion at the distal anastomosis of a saphenous vein graft (SVG) to the posterior descending artery (PDA). A: 3D volume rendering reconstruction showing an inferior view of the heart in which the anastomosis of the graft is seen (An). B: Detailed 3D image of the distal anastomosis of the SVG, in which a stenosis is observed (yellow arrow). C: MIP image showing the stenosis at the anastomotic site. PL: posterolateral branch of the right coronary artery.

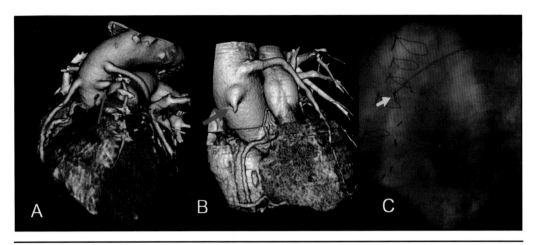

FIGURE 4.81 Examples of saphenous vein grafts occluded at their origin. A and B: 3D volume rendering reconstructions from two different patients showing the typical image in the ascending aortic wall resembling a stump (red arrows), indicating the lack of progression of the contrast beyond the occlusion site, this preventing the visualization of the rest of the graft, at the present setting of window width/level. C: Invasive coronary angiogram corresponding to the patient shown in B, confirming the graft occlusion (yellow arrow).

positive remodeling that enlarges the whole diameter of the vessel. This explains why these lesions may pass undetected by conventional angiography[36], their adequate invasive assessment requiring IVUS studies. The promising results of comparison between MDCT and IVUS[2,40,56,57] allow consideration of MDCT as a useful tool in the noninvasive detection of potentially threatening coronary artery lesions.

The technique still has, however, some limitations in this sense. Although recent equipments offer spatial resolution at the submillimetric level (0.5 mm) which is adequate for a morphological assessment of lesions, it does not permit visualization of important (though very small) structures, such as the fibrous cap of the lesions[44]. The use of Hounsfield units value as a surrogate method for the identification of plaque components is also limited by the heterogeneous nature of lesions themselves; the

attenuation coefficient of thrombotic material into the vessel lumen, for instance, is close to that exhibited by adipose plaques[44]. In addition, the acquisition technique for a proper classification of a lesion has not yet been standardized, and MDCT can only provide a mere indication of the predominant component.

The description of an atherosclerotic lesion by MDCT is, in summary, highly informative, as it includes its morphological features, degree of remodeling of the vessel wall, presence of calcification, and attenuation properties of the plaque itself, this constituting an approach to the recognition of its main tissue component[43].

4.2.2.4 Non-atherosclerotic coronary artery disease

Besides congenital anomalies of the origin of coronary arteries (discussed in Chapter 2),

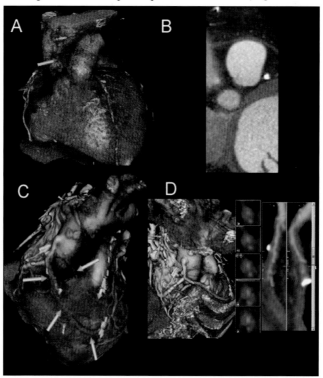

FIGURE 4.82 Visualization of the distal course of coronary saphenous vein grafts occluded at the proximal site; images are obtained from reconstructions in which the window width/level (W/L) has been optimized in order to show not only the contrast but also other less dense structures, such as vessels filled with atherothrombotic or fibrotic content. A and B: 3D volume rendering (A) and curved MPR reconstruction (B) of one of the occluded grafts (red arrows). Note the low density of the occluded graft, which is clearly different from a normal graft filled with contrast (see Figure 4.69). C: 3D volume rendering showing two saphenous vein grafts, both of them occluded. D: Curved MPR reconstruction of one of these grafts shows progression of the contrast in the proximal segment followed by a sharp density reduction.

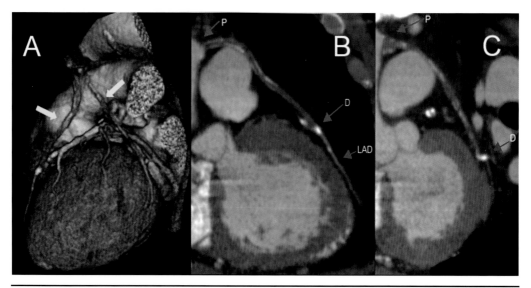

FIGURE 4.83 A: 3D volume rendering reconstruction of two saphenous vein coronary grafts to the left anterior descending artery and marginal obtuse branch, both occluded at their proximal site (yellow arrows). These grafts show a significantly lower density than that of the rest of the vessels filled with contrast, although their course can still be depicted due to the presence of a calcified graft wall. B and C: Curved MPR reconstructions of the entire course of both grafts, from the proximal (P) to the distal (D) end; image in B clearly shows a decreased density of the graft when compared with the distal native vessel (LAD), due to the lack of contrast within the graft.

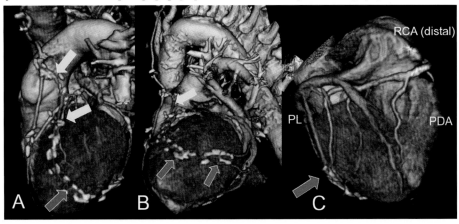

FIGURE 4.84 Competitive flow of a radial artery graft with proximal anastomosis to an internal mammary artery graft and distally to a posterolateral branch of the right coronary artery. A: 3D reconstruction showing a gradual decrease of the graft density from its proximal site (yellow arrows) to its distal portion (red arrows). B: The distal portion of the graft is barely seen (red arrows), and only the metallic clips are distinguished. C: Distal anastomosis of the radial graft (red arrow) to the posterolateral branch of the right coronary artery, and distal vessel of the posterolateral branch proximal to the bypass anastomosis. This distal vessel shows a large diameter without any critical stenosis, resulting in competitive flow.

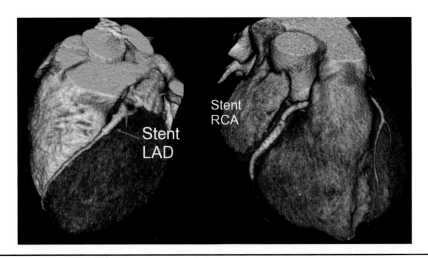

FIGURE 4.85 3D volume rendering reconstructions showing coronary stents in the left anterior descending (LAD) and right coronary artery (RCA). Note the striking appearance of the stent, with the metallic mesh shown as a cylindric structure apparently protruding beyond the limits of the vessel. The vessel distal to the stent is clearly visualized, indicating stent patency.

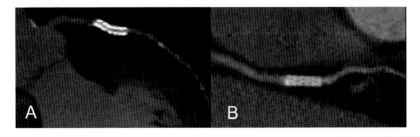

FIGURE 4.86 A: Stent placed in the middle segment of the left anterior descending artery. Curved MPR reconstruction shows the marked partial volume artifact due to the metallic component of the stent. It is not possible to rule out an in-stent stenotic lesion. B: Stent placed in the distal right coronary artery clearly showing its metallic structure which does not allow evaluation of its lumen. However, in both cases, the vessel distal to the stent is clearly visualized, this suggesting stent patency.

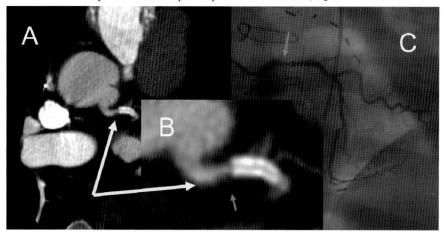

FIGURE 4.87 A: Pre-stent lesion of the circumflex artery. B: Detailed image of the lesion. The lesion proximal to the stent may be detected in spite that the metallic artifact impedes evaluation of the in-stent lumen. C: Image of the lesion in the invasive coronary angiogram.

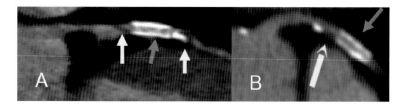

FIGURE 4.88 A: Significant stenotic lesions in the proximal and distal sites (yellow arrows) of a coronary stent (red arrow). The proximal lesion is mainly fibrolipidic while the distal one is markedly calcified. B: Nonsignificant stenotic lesion in the proximal site of a coronary stent.

there are a number of non-atherosclerotic abnormalities (also mainly congenital), that can be depicted with great anatomical detail by MDCT.

4.2.2.4.1 Arteriovenous coronary fistula

Detected in 0.1–0.2% of invasive coronary angiographies, coronary fistulae most commonly originate from the right coronary artery and drain into the right ventricle (40%), right atria (25%), or even the pulmonary artery (17%)[69,70]. Coronary fistulae may course clinically asymptomatic (50%) or may cause congestive heart failure, angina, or be the substrate for a case of infective endocarditis. Fistulae can be detected by echocardiography[71,72], although their precise study requires the practice of an invasive angiography which provides appropriate information on the origin and drainage of the involved vessel. Angiography is, however, somewhat limited in determining

the relationship of the fistulous vessel with surrounding structures.

The appropriate resolution of MDCT, particularly with multiplanar and 3D reconstruction, may provide adequate information on all anatomical aspects of coronary fistulae[73–75] (Figure 4.93), which is highly useful in cases where a surgical approach is planned.

4.2.2.4.2 Myocardial bridge

This anomaly is described to be present in nearly one third of adults, although it is detected by angiography in less than 5% of individuals[76]. A particularly high prevalence of myocardial bridge has been reported among patients with hypertrophic cardiomyopathy and cardiac transplant recipients. The most frequent location of muscular bridges is the middle segment of the LAD coronary artery, particularly when there are two parallel LAD vessels, in which case one of them usually presents with some intramyocardial course. The length of a bridged coronary

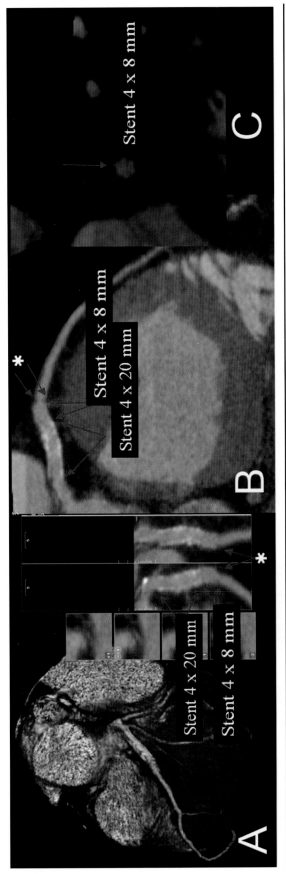

FIGURE 4.89 Stents 4-mm in diameter placed in the proximal segment of the left anterior descending artery. A: 3D and MPR showing that an appropriate visualization of the lumen is possible in cases of large diameter stents, excluding significant stenotic lesions. B: Curved MPR reconstruction showing a mild residual non calcified lesion (asterisk) at the distal edge of the shorter stent (4 × 8 mm). C: Transverse section of the 4 × 8 mm stent that allows visualization of the intravascular lumen and the hexagonal structure of the stent mesh.

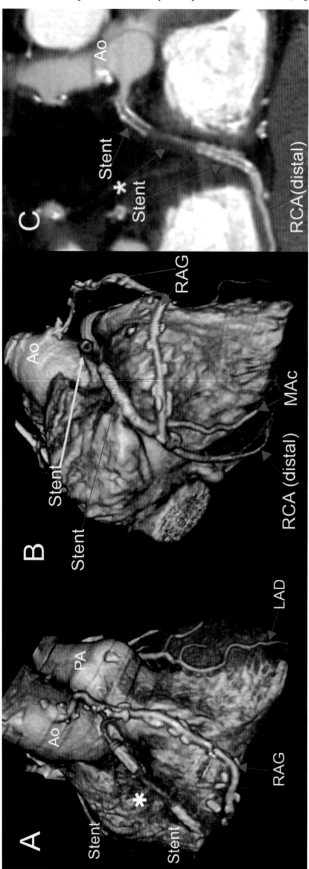

FIGURE 4.90 Images from a patient with two occluded coronary stents in the proximal and middle segments of the right coronary artery (RCA) and a subsequent surgical revascularization with a radial artery graft (RAG). A: 3D volume rendering showing showing poor lumen density (asterisk) of the middle segment of the native RCA (between both stents) indicating vessel occlusion. B: Caudal view showing the poor lumen density in the proximal stent (yellow arrow), suggesting stent occlusion. C: Curved MPR showing reduced signal density of the RCA from its origin involving both stents and the native segment in between (asterisk), this indicating vessel occlusion; observe high density at the lumen of the distal RCA indicating patency, the flow being provided by the RAG. Ao: aorta; MAc: marginal acute branch; PA: pulmonary artery.

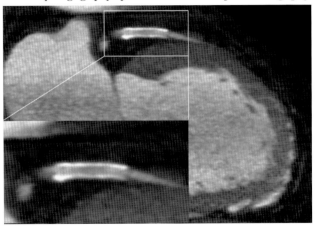

FIGURE 4.91 A 4-mm diameter stent placed in the left anterior descending artery. The large diameter of the stent allows an adequate visualization of the lumen ruling out, in this case, any significant in-stent lesion.

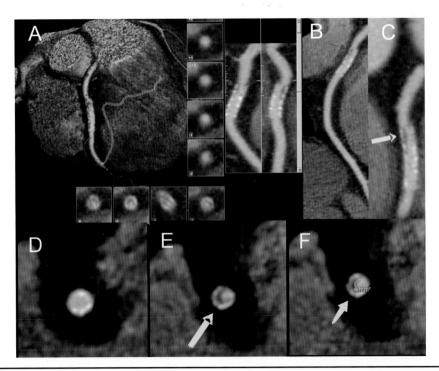

FIGURE 4.92 Images from a patient with an in-stent coronary lesion in a 4-mm diameter stent placed in the proximal segment of the right coronary artery. A: 3D volume rendering and curved MPR showing the stent lumen in 2 orthogonal sections of the vessel and in different transversal sections; an area of reduced lumen density is observed (red arrows) suggesting in-stent lesion. B: Curved MPR showing the whole vessel length. C: Detailed image of the lesion (yellow arrow). D: Cross-sectional view of the stent at its distal site showing absence of lesion at this level. E: Cross-sectional view of the proximal end of the stent showing the lesion (arrow). F: Measurement of the luminal area of the vessel at the site of the lesion.

artery segment is between 10–30 mm, being the thickness of the muscular bridge between 1–10 mm.

The diagnosis of a myocardial bridge over a coronary artery is performed at the angiography by visualizing a "milking" effect due to a compression during systole of the bridged segment. This abnormality may lead to myocardial ischemia, particularly in those cases with thick muscular bridges. Thin bridges may pass undetected to angiography due to a mild milking effect. The high resolution

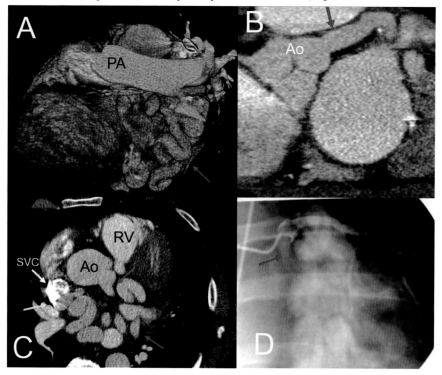

FIGURE 4.93 Coronary fistula involving the left coronary artery. A: 3D volume rendering provides detailed anatomy of the course of the fistula (arrow). B: Curved MPR showing the origin of the fistulous coronary artery in the aortic root (Ao). C: Axial image showing the course of the fistula (red arrows) and its drainage in the superior vena cava (SVC) (yellow arrow). D: Invasive coronary angiogram; although proving the presence of a coronary fistula (arrow), the angiography provides limited information on its anatomical relationships. PA: pulmonary artery; RV: right ventricle.

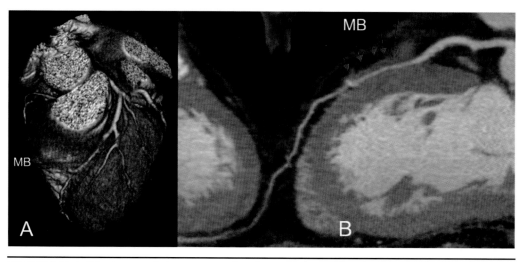

FIGURE 4.94 A: 3D volume rendering reconstruction of a myocardial bridge (MB) located in the middle segment of the left anterior descending artery. B: Curved MPR reconstruction showing the bridged coronary segment within the myocardial wall (red arrows).

of MDCT imaging allows the detection of myocardial bridges[77], whatever their thickness (Figures 4.63, 4.94 and 4.95). The visualization

of the milking effect, however, is usually not adequate by this technique, provided the limited temporal resolution of cine loop images.

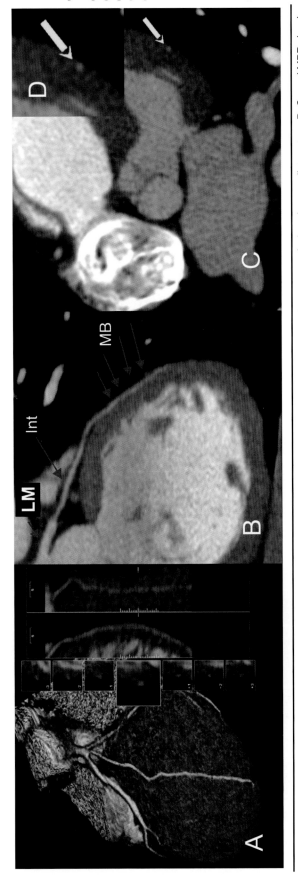

FIGURE 4.95 A: 3D volume rendering reconstruction of a myocardial coronary bridge that involves the middle and distal segments of a long intermediate artery. B: Curved MPR showing the shallow tunneled coronary segment (MB). C: Axial image that clearly shows the intramyocardial course of the vessel (yellow arrow) along the myocardial lateral wall. D: Detailed image of the intramyocardial course of the artery on the axial view. LM: left main; Int: intermediate artery.

4.2.2.4.3 Coronary artery ectasy and aneurysm

An increase in the diameter of a coronary artery segment over 1.5 times the one of an adjacent healthy segment of the vessel is considered an abnormal dilatation[78]. When extense epicardial portions of the coronary arteries are involved, the term ectasy is applied, while the term aneurysm implies a localized dilatation of a vessel. The etiology in both cases is atherosclerotic in nearly 50% of patients[79–82], and due to inflammatory diseases (Kawasaki) or congenital in the rest.

Coronary ectasy usually involves the RCA and is found in 1–3% of patients with obstructive atherosclerotic coronary artery disease, although its clinical significance is controversial; while 70% of patients present with data on inducible myocardial ischemia are not responsive to nitroglycerin, ectasic coronary arteries do not seem to have an impact on the incidence of myocardial infarction or on survival rates[79,80].

When isolate, a coronary aneurysm is frequently associated with atherosclerotic disease[83,84], usually involving the LAD coronary artery. In cases due to Kawasaki's disease, coronary aneurysms can be large[85] and multiple. While frequently asymptomatic, coronary aneurysms may cause local thrombosis with distal embolization or rupture of the vessel wall, a rare and unpredictable complication.

Coronary ectasy and aneurysm are usually incidental findings[79] at angiography, and can also be very well depicted by MDCT[86] (Figures 4.96–4.98).

4.3 Role of Noninvasive Coronary Angiography by MDCT in Clinical Practice

The diagnostic accuracy of MDCT coronary angiography is fairly high but not exactly comparable to invasive angiography, which cannot be substituted by MDCT when indicated[20]. On the other hand, there are no established guides at present for the clinical application of noninvasive coronary angiography[87,88].

Nevertheless, MDCT has a potentially relevant role in clinical practice, particularly in those patients not considered for an invasive angiography as an immediate diagnostic choice, but in whom there is still concern of the presence of a coronary artery disease. Useful in this sense is the high negative predictive value of the technique[2–4] that permits ruling out the disease accurately. Thus, groups of patients that could benefit from its use are those with nonspecific symptoms and inconclusive provocative tests, those in whom it is mandatory to rule out coronary disease before valvular cardiac surgery, or more simply, those asymptomatic individuals with a prominently high-risk factor profile (Figure 4.35). The technique is also of consideration in patients with overt coronary artery disease under a stable situation who have not been previously submitted to invasive angiography, in whom MDCT usually provides important morphological information on the responsible artery (Figure 4.66). The information from MDCT may be, in these cases,

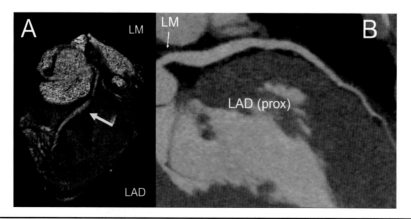

FIGURE 4.96 A: 3D volume rendering in a case of coronary ectasia of the middle segment of the left anterior descending artery (LAD) (yellow arrow). B: Curved MPR from another patient, in this case with a coronary ectasia involving the proximal segment of the LAD (red arrow). Observe that, contrary to the normal situation, the diameter of the LAD is larger than that of the left main (LM).

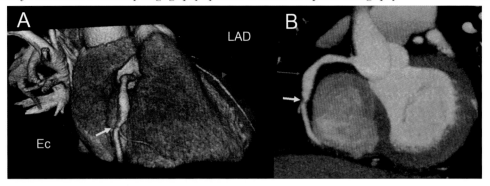

FIGURE 4.97 A: 3D volume rendering showing coronary ectasia (Ec) at the middle segment of the right coronary artery; a stenotic lesion is also observed in the distal end of the ectasic segment (yellow arrow). B: MIP image clearly defines the extension of the coronary ectasia (red arrow) and the severity of the stenotic lesion distal to it (yellow arrow).

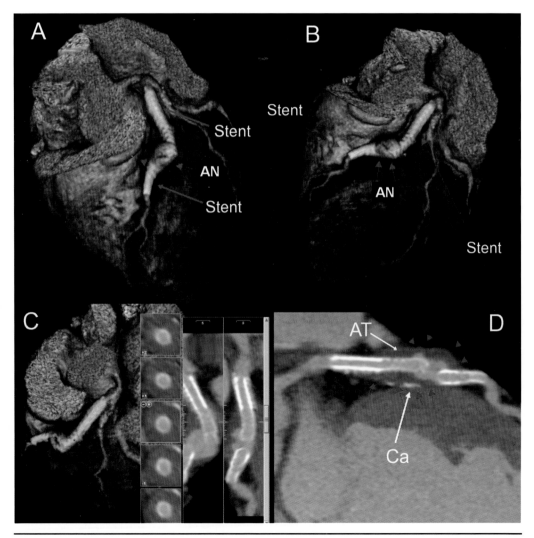

FIGURE 4.98 A and B: 3D volume rendering showing a coronary aneurysm in the middle segment of the left anterior descending artery, located between two stents. C: Curved MPR showing patency of the stents. D: Curved MPR showing the wall of the aneurysm (red arrows), its low density atherothrombotic contents (AT), and some foci of parietal calcium (Ca).

highly valuable in terms of stratification and prognosis, together with provocative tests. Finally, also in those patients repeatedly submitted to catheterization, particularly with coronary artery grafts, who present with recurrent anginal symptoms, MDCT can be an alternative to non-invasively evaluate the state of native vessels and the bypass grafts[89]. When a further intervention is planned, the anatomical information on the thoracic structures provided by MDCT[90,91] (Figure 4.67) can also be very helpful for the surgical approach.

References

1. Leschka, S., et al. Accuracy of MSCT coronary angiography with 64-slice technology: first experience. *Eur Heart J*, 2005, 26, 1482–7.

2. Leber, A.W., et al. Quantification of obstructive and nonobstructive coronary lesions by 64-slice computed tomography: a comparative study with quantitative coronary angiography and intravascular ultrasound. *J Am Coll Cardiol*, 2005, 46, 147–54.

3. Raff, G.L., et al. Diagnostic accuracy of noninvasive coronary angiography using 64-slice spiral computed tomography. *J Am Coll Cardiol*, 2005, 46, 552–7.

4. Mollet, N.R., et al. High-resolution spiral computed tomography coronary angiography in patients referred for diagnostic conventional coronary angiography. *Circulation*, 2005, 112, 2318–23.

5. Ropers, D., et al. Investigation of aortocoronary artery bypass grafts by multislice spiral computed tomography with electrocardiographic-gated image reconstruction. *Am J Cardiol*, 2001, 88, 792–5.

6. Nieman, K., et al. Evaluation of patients after coronary artery bypass surgery: CT angiographic assessment of grafts and coronary arteries. *Radiology*, 2003, 229, 749–56.

7. Dewey, M., et al. Isotropic half-millimeter angiography of coronary artery bypass grafts with 16-slice computed tomography. *Ann Thorac Surg*, 2004, 77, 800–4.

8. Martuscelli, E., et al. Evaluation of venous and arterial conduit patency by 16-slice spiral computed tomography. *Circulation*, 2004, 110, 3234–8.

9. Schlosser, T., et al. Noninvasive visualization of coronary artery bypass grafts using 16-detector row computed tomography. *J Am Coll Cardiol*, 2004, 44, 1224–9.

10. Song, M.H., et al. Multidetector computed tomography versus coronary angiogram in evaluation of coronary artery bypass grafts. *Ann Thorac Surg*, 2005, 79, 585–8.

11. Trigo, A., et al. Non-invasive assessment of coronary artery bypass grafts by computed tomography: comparison with conventional coronary angiography. *Rev Esp Cardiol*, 2005, 58, 807–14.

12. Nieman, K., et al. Coronary angiography with multi-slice computed tomography. *Lancet*, 2001, 357, 599–603.

13. Knez, A., et al. Usefulness of multislice spiral computed tomography angiography for determination of coronary artery stenoses. *Am J Cardiol*, 2001, 88, 1191–4.

14. Achenbach, S., et al. Detection of coronary artery stenoses by contrast-enhanced, retrospectively electrocardiographically-gated, multislice spiral computed tomography. *Circulation*, 2001, 103, 2535–8.

15. Nieman, K., et al. Usefulness of multislice computed tomography for detecting obstructive coronary artery disease. *Am J Cardiol*, 2002, 89, 913–8.

16. Vogl, T.J., et al. Techniques for the detection of coronary atherosclerosis: multi-detector row CT coronary angiography. *Radiology*, 2002, 223, 212–20.

17. Kuettner, A., et al. Diagnostic accuracy of multidetector computed tomography coronary angiography in patients with angiographically proven coronary artery disease. *J Am Coll Cardiol*, 2004, 43, 831–9.

18. Nieman, K., et al. Reliable noninvasive coronary angiography with fast submillimeter multislice spiral computed tomography. *Circulation*, 2002, 107, 2051–4.

19. Ropers, D., et al. Detection of coronary artery stenoses with thin-slices multidetector row spiral computed tomography and multiplanar reconstruction. *Circulation*, 2003, 107, 664–6.

20. Leta, R., et al. Non-invasive coronary angiography with 16 multidetector-row spiral computed tomography: a comparative study with invasive coronary angiography. *Rev Esp Cardiol*, 2004, 57, 217–24.

21. Mollet, N.R., et al. Multislice spiral computed tomography coronary angiography in patients

with stable angina pectoris. *J Am Coll Cardiol*, 2004, 43, 2265–70.

22. Hoffmann, U., et al. Predictive value of 16-slice multidetector spiral computed tomography to detect significant obstructive coronary artery disease in patients at high risk for coronary artery disease: patient-versus segment-based analysis. *Circulation*, 2004, 110, 2638–43.

23. Kuettner, A., et al. Diagnostic accuracy of noninvasive coronary imaging using 16-detector slice spiral computed tomography with 188 ms temporal resolution. *J Am Coll Cardiol*, 2005, 45, 123–7.

24. Hoffmann, M.H., et al. Noninvasive coronary angiography with multislice computed tomography. *JAMA*, 2005, 293, 2471–8.

25. Nakanishi, T., et al. Pitfalls in 16-detector row CT of the coronary arteries. *Radiographics*, 2005, 25, 425–38.

26. Friesinger, G.C., and J.M. Perry, Jr. Coronary arteriography: indications and pitfalls. *Cardiovasc Clin*, 1975, 6, 265–81.

27. Yamashita, T., A. Colombo, and J.M. Tobis. Limitations of coronary angiography compared with intravascular ultrasound: implications for coronary interventions. *Prog Cardiovasc Dis*, 1999, 42, 91–138.

28. Mintz, G.S., et al. Atherosclerosis in angiographically "normal" coronary artery reference segments: an intravascular ultrasound study with clinical correlations. *J Am Coll Cardiol*, 1995, 25, 1479–85.

29. Johnston, P.W., S. Fort, and E.A. Cohen. Noncritical disease of the left main coronary artery: limitations of angiography and the role of intravascular ultrasound. *Can J Cardiol*, 1999, 15, 297–302.

30. Hong, M.K., et al. Limitations of angiography for analyzing coronary atherosclerosis progresion or regression. *Ann Intern Med*, 1994, 121, 348–54.

31. Mintz, G.S., et al. Limitations of angiography in the assessment of plaque distribution in coronary artery disease: a systematic study of target lesion eccentricity in 1446 lesions. *Circulation*, 1996, 93, 924–31.

32. Katritsis, D., and M. Webb-Peploe. Limitations of coronary angiography: an underestimated problem? *Clin Cardiol*, 1991, 14, 20–4.

33. Botas, J. Assessment and therapeutic guideline of intermediate coronary lesions in the catheterization laboratory. *Rev Esp Cardiol*, 2003, 56, 1218–30.

34. Nissen, S.E., and P. Yock. Intravascular ultrasound: novel pathophysiological insights and current clinical applications. *Circulation*, 2001, 103, 604–16.

35. Lee, D.Y., et al. Effect of intracoronary ultrasound imaging on clinical decision making. *Am Heart J*, 1995, 129, 1084–93.

36. Caussin, C., et al. Coronary plaque burden detected by multislice computed tomography after acute myocardial infarction with near-normal coronary arteries by angiography. *Am J Cardiol*, 2003, 92, 849–52.

37. Leber, A.W., et al. Accuracy of multidetector spiral computed tomography in identifying and differentiating the composition of coronary atherosclerotic plaques: a comparative study with intracoronary ultrasound. *J Am Coll Cardiol*, 2004, 43, 1241–7.

38. Schoenhagen, P., et al. Non-invasive assessment of plaque morphology and remodeling in mildly stenotic coronary segments: comparison of 16-slice computed tomography and intravascular ultrasound. *Coron Artery Dis*, 2003, 14, 459–62.

39. Achenbach, S., et al. Detection of calcified and noncalcified coronary atherosclerotic plaque by contrast-enhanced, submillimeter multidetector spiral computed tomography: a segment-based comparison with intravascular ultrasound. *Circulation*, 2004, 109, 14–7.

40. Achenbach, S., et al. Assessment of coronary remodeling in stenotic and nonstenotic coronary atherosclerotic lesions by multidetector spiral computed tomography. *J Am Coll Cardiol*, 2004, 43, 842–7.

41. Lawler, L.P., H.K. Pannu, and E.K. Fishman. MDCT evaluation of the coronary arteries, 2004: how we do it-data acquisition, post-processing, display, and interpretation. *Am J Roentgenol*, 2005, 184, 1402–12.

42. Schragin, J.G., et al. Non-cardiac findings on coronary electron beam computed tomography scanning. *J Thorac Imaging*, 2004, 19, 82–6.

43. Prokop, M., and A.J. Van der Molen. *Spiral and Multislice Computed Tomography of the Body, 1st ed.* Stuttgart: Thieme Verlag, 2003, 804–7.

44. Schroeder, S., et al. Reliability of differentiating human coronary plaque morphology using contrast-enhanced multislice spiral computed tomography: a comparison with histology. *J Comput Assist Tomogr*, 2004, 28, 449–54.

45. de Feyter, P., et al. Noninvasive visualisation of coronary atherosclerosis with multislice computed tomography. *Cardiovasc Radiat Med*, 2004, 5, 49–56.

46. Gerber, T.C., et al. Current results and new developments of coronary angiography with use of contrast-enhanced computed tomography of the heart. *Mayo Clin Proc*, 2002, 77, 55–71.

47. van Ooijen, P.M., et al. Coronary artery imaging with multidetector CT: visualization issues. *Radiographics*, 2003, 23, e16.

48. Bache, R.J. Vasodilator reserve: a functional assessment of coronary health. *Circulation*, 1998, 98, 1257–60.

49. Brown, B.G., E.L. Bolson, and H.T. Dodge. Dynamic mechanisms in human coronary stenosis. *Circulation*, 1984, 70, 917–22.

50. Gould, K.L., K. Lipscomb, and G.W. Hamilton. Physiologic basis for assessing critical coronary stenosis. Instantaneous flow response and regional distribution during coronary hyperemia as measures of coronary flow reserve. *Am J Cardiol*, 1974, 33, 87–94.

51. Keane, D., et al. Comparative validation of quantitative coronary angiography systems: Results and implications from a multicenter study using a standardized approach. *Circulation*, 1995, 91, 2174–83.

52. Herrington, D.M., M. Siebes, and G.D. Walford. Sources of error in quantitative coronary angiography. *Cathet Cardiovasc Diagn*, 1993, 29, 314–21.

53. Takagi, A., et al. Clinical potential of intravascular ultrasound for physiological assessment of coronary stenosis: relationship between quantitative ultrasound tomography and pressure-derived fractional flow reserve. *Circulation*, 1999, 100, 250–5.

54. Jasti, V., et al. Correlations between fractional flow reserve and intravascular ultrasound in patients with an ambiguous left main coronary artery stenosis. *Circulation*, 2004, 110, 2831–6.

55. Hermiller, J.B., et al. Unrecognized left main coronary artery disease in patients undergoing interventional procedures. *Am J Cardiol*, 1993, 71, 173–176.

56. Komatsu, S., et al. Detection of coronary plaque by computed tomography with a novel plaque analysis system, 'Plaque Map', and comparison with intravascular ultrasound and angioscopy. *Circ J*, 2005, 69, 72–7.

57. Caussin, C., et al. Comparison of lumens of intermediate coronary stenosis using 16-slice computed tomography versus intravascular ultrasound. *Am J Cardiol*, 2005, 96, 524–8.

58. Mollet, N.R., et al. Value of preprocedure multislice computed tomographic coronary angiog-raphy to predict the outcome of percutaneous recanalization of chronic total occlusions. *Am J Cardiol*, 2005, 95, 240–3.

59. Chiurlia, E., et al. Follow-up of coronary artery bypass graft patency by multislice computed tomography. *Am J Cardiol*, 2005, 95, 1094–7.

60. Marano, R., et al. Pictorial review of coronary artery bypass graft at multidetector row CT. *Chest*, 2005, 127, 1371–7.

61. Schuijf, J.D., et al. Feasibility of assessment of coronary stent patency using 16-slice computed tomography. *Am J Cardiol*, 2004, 94, 427–30.

62. Maintz, D., et al. Imaging of coronary artery stents using multislice computed tomography: in vitro evaluation. *Eur Radiol*, 2003, 13, 830–5.

63. Cademartiri, F., et al. Usefulness of multislice computed tomographic coronary angiography to assess in-stent restenosis. *Am J Cardiol*, 2005, 96, 799–802.

64. Gaspar, T., et al. Diagnosis of coronary in-stent restenosis with multidetector row spiral computed tomography. *J Am Coll Cardiol*, 2005, 46, 1573–9.

65. Gilard, M., et al. Noninvasive assessment of left main coronary stent patency with 16-slice computed tomography. *Am J Cardiol*, 2005, 95, 110–2.

66. Stary, H.C. Natural history and histological classification of atherosclerotic lesions: An update. *Arterioscler Thromb Vasc Biol*, 2000, 20, 1177–8.

67. Virmani, R., et al. Lessons from sudden coronary death: a comprehensive morphological classification scheme for atherosclerotic atherosclerotic lesions. *Arterioscler Thromb Vasc Biol*, 2000, 20, 1262–75.

68. Libby, P., and P. Theroux. Pathophysiology of coronary artery disease. *Circulation*, 2005, 111, 3481–8.

69. Lipiec, P., et al. Right coronary artery-to-right ventricle fistula complicating percutaneoustransluminal angioplasty: case report and review of the literature. *J Am Soc Echocardiogr*, 2004, 17, 280–3.

70. Darwazah, A.K., I.H. Hussein, and M.H. Hawari. Congenital circumflex coronary arteriovenous fistula with aneurysmal termination in the pulmonary artery. *Tex Heart Inst J*, 2005, 32, 56–9.

71. Yilmaz, R., R. Demirbag, and M. Gur. Echocardiographic diagnosis of a right coronary

artery-coronary sinus fistula. *Int J Cardiovasc Imaging*, 2005, 21, 649–54.

72. Iida, R., et al. Identification of the site of drainage of left main coronary artery to right atrium fistula with intraoperative transesophageal echocardiography. *J Cardiothorac Vasc Anesth*, 2005, 19, 777–80.

73. Tan, K.T., R. Chamberlain-Webber, and G. Mc-Gann. Characterisation of coronary artery fistula by multi-slice computed tomography. *Int J Cardiol*, 2005.

74. Chang, D.S., et al. MDCT of Left Anterior Descending Coronary Artery to Main Pulmonary Artery Fistula. *Am J Roentgenol*, 2005, 185, 1258–60.

75. Soon, K.H., et al. Giant single coronary system with coronary cameral fistula diagnosed on MSCT. *Int J Cardiol*, 2006, 106, 276–8.

76. Mohlenkamp, S., et al. Update on myocardial bridging. *Circulation*, 2002, 106, 2616–22.

77. Goitein, O., and J.M. Lacomis. Myocardial bridging: noninvasive diagnosis with multidetector CT. *J Comput Assist Tomogr*, 2005, 29, 238–40.

78. Kosar, F., et al. Effect of ectasia size or the ectasia ratio on the thrombosis in myocardial infarction frame count in patients with isolated coronary artery ectasia. *Heart Vessels*, 2005, 20, 199–202.

79. Hartnell, G.G., B.M. Parnell, and R.B. Pridie. Coronary artery ectasia. Its prevalence and clinical significance in 4993 patients. *Br Heart J*, 1985, 54, 392–5.

80. Braunwald, E., D.P. Zipes, and P. Libby. *Heart Disease: a textbook of cardiovascular Medicine, 6th ed.* Philadelphia: WB Saunders, 2001.

81. Tunick, P.A., et al. Discrete atherosclerotic coronary artery aneurysms: A study of 20 patients. *J Am Coll Cardiol*, 1990, 15, 279–82.

82. Okmen, E., et al. Left main coronary artery aneurysm associated with extensive coronary arterial calcification: case report and review. *Int J Cardiovasc Imaging*, 2004, 20, 231–5.

83. Abbate, A., et al. Left main coronary artery aneurysm: a case report and review of the literature. *Ital Heart J*, 2001, 2, 711–4.

84. Pineda, G.E., et al. Large atherosclerotic left main coronary aneurysm—a case report and review of the literature. *Angiology*, 2001, 52, 501–4.

85. Rozo, J.C., et al. Kawasaki disease in the adult: a case report and review of the literature. *Tex Heart Inst J*, 2004, 31, 160–4.

86. Kanamaru, H., et al. Assessment of coronary artery abnormalities by multislice spiral computed tomography in adolescents and young adults with Kawasaki disease. *Am J Cardiol*, 2005, 95, 522–5.

87. Sechtem, U., and M. Vöhringer. The clinical role of "non-invasive" coronary angiography by multidetector spiral computed tomography: yet to be defined. *Eur Heart J*, 2005, 26, 1942–4.

88. J de Feyter, P., and B.W. Meijboom. Multislice computed tomography coronary angiography: Prime time? *Rev Esp Cardiol*, 2005, 58, 1253–7.

89. Frazier, A.A., et al. Coronary artery bypass grafts: assessment with multidetector CT in the early and late postoperative settings. *Radiographics*, 2005, 25, 881–96.

90. Gasparovic, H., et al. Three-dimensional computed tomographic imaging in planning the surgical approach for redo cardiac surgery after coronary revascularization. *Eur J Cardiothorac Surg*, 2005, 28, 244–9.

91. Gilkeson, R.C., A.H. Markowitz, and L. Ciancibello. Multisection CT evaluation of the reoperative cardiac surgery patient. *Radiographics*, 2003, 23, S3–17.

Morphological and Functional Assessment of Heart Chambers by MDCT

5

GUILLEM PONS-LLADÓ

Noninvasive coronary angiography constitutes the most important contribution of multidetector computed tomography (MDCT) to the diagnostic field in cardiology. There is, however, a large amount of data contained in the thoracic volume acquired during the exam which can provide interesting additional information, particularly on cardiovascular morphology and function.

An advantageous aspect of MDCT in this respect is that all these data are available from the single initial acquisition, not requiring a particular strategy, in contrast to echocardiography (ECHO) or to cardiovascular magnetic resonance (CMR). This makes MDCT a unique imaging technique, as this information can be selectively retrieved in each case from the same volume used for the assessment of coronary arteries.

5.1 Assessment of Ventricular Volume and Function

Data on volume and function, particularly of the left ventricle, constitute important clinical information in all patients with heart disease. While a number of other imaging methods provide accurate data on these parameters and can be applied in clinical routine, MDCT estimations are valuable in those patients with proven or suspected ischemic heart disease who are submitted to a noninvasive coronary angiography study[1].

The analysis of ventricular volume and function is performed from multiplanar reformations of the retrospectively ECG-gated data set obtained for coronary artery imaging. Reconstructions of phase images are performed throughout the whole cardiac cycle in 5% increasing steps, 20 heart phases being thus obtained that can be displayed as a loop in cine format. Temporal resolution varies between 100 and 250 msec., depending on the heart rate of the patient and the reconstruction algorithm[2].

The obtention of planes aligned with the axes of the heart itself is important for an adequate analysis of global and, particularly, regional left ventricular function. These orientations can be easily obtained starting from the actual axial plane, where an oblique sagittal orientation transecting the apex and the base of the left ventricle (Figure 5.1A) gives a longitudinal vertical plane containing the two

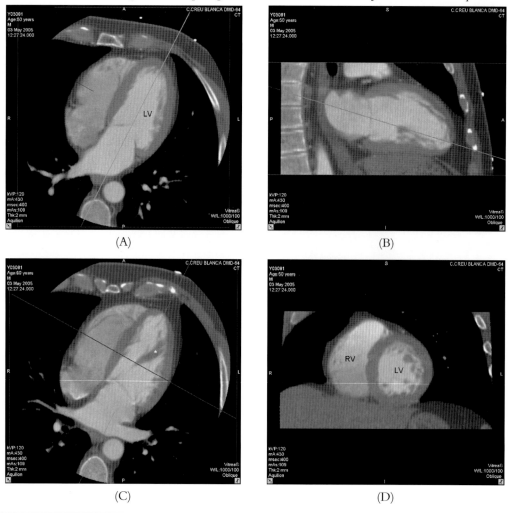

(A)   (B)

(C)   (D)

FIGURE 5.1 Method for the obtention of longitudinal and short-axis planes of the ventricles through multiplanar reconstruction. (A) Axial plane including the apex and the mitral valve plane of the left ventricle (LV); a line transecting these regions indicates the orientation of a vertical longitudinal plane of the left ventricle; (B) 2-chamber view obtained from the orientation in (A); a new line containing the base and the apex of the ventricle is traced; (C) Horizontal longitudinal plane (4-chamber view) resulting from the orientation in (B); the anterior papillary muscle (asterisk) is frequently included in this view; a line indicates the orientation of a short-axis plane; (D) Plane resulting from the orientation shown in (C), where both the right (RV) and left (LV) ventricles are included.

left heart chambers (Figure 5.1B), where a new orientation using the same reference points will render a longitudinal horizontal plane of the heart (4-chamber) (Figure 5.1C). From these longitudinal views of the heart, a series of short-axis planes can be obtained (Figure 5.1D).

The operator may visually select for calculations the end-diastolic and end-systolic frames by reviewing the reconstructed phases in any of these orientations. Longitudinal views allow for a fast calculation of left ventricular volumes based on an area-length method (Figure 5.2), while an estimation of the true left ventricular volume from the whole 3D dataset is also

possible by means of dedicated software analysis packages able to detect the endocardial border of the ventricle (Figure 5.3).

Measurements of left ventricular parameters with MDCT have been correlated with those from CMR[3] showing good correlations, although with a mild overestimation for end-diastolic and end-systolic volumes, and excellent agreement with respect to ejection fraction. A relative limitation of MDCT in the estimation of ejection fraction is the obtention of a truly end-systolic frame, provided that the time interval where the minimal left ventricular volume is maintained in the normal

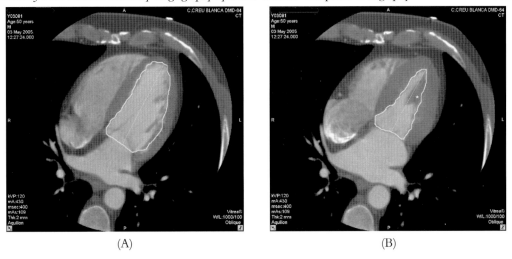

(A) (B)

FIGURE 5.2 Diastolic (A) and systolic (B) frames from a 4-chamber view where endocardial areas and axis of the left ventricle have been determined for the calculation of volumes by means of an area-length method. Note that the anterior papillary muscle (asterisk) is excluded from the calculation of the systolic area.

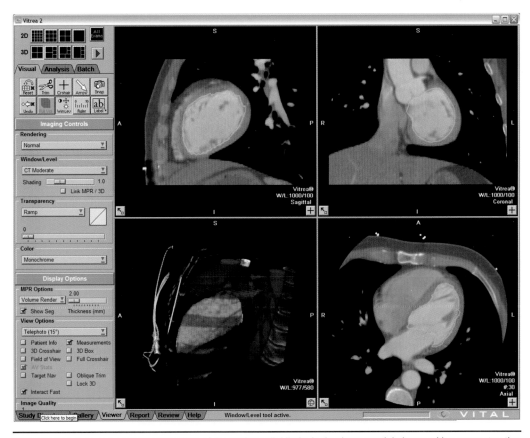

FIGURE 5.3 Automatic contour detection of the endocardial limits in the three spatial planes with a reconstruction of the left ventricular volume (bottom left panel) as performed on a dedicated workstation.

heart may be shorter than the actual temporal resolution of current MDCT systems[4]. Further improvements in temporal resolution will probably refine the accuracy of volume calculations by this technique. Measurements of right ventricular volumes and ejection fraction have also been attempted, in this case using electron-beam computed tomography[5], and proven to closely correlate with measures from CMR, despite a small overestimation of both end-diastolic and end-systolic volumes.

The analysis of cine loop formats in any of the mentioned planes allows for a qualitative assessment of regional left ventricular function (Figure 5.4) and the identification of areas of

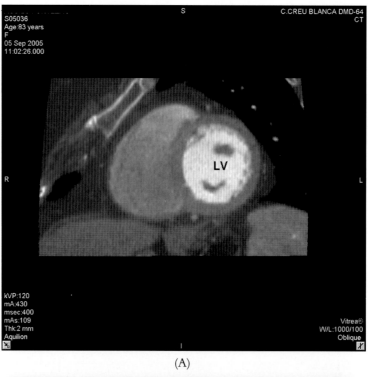

(A)

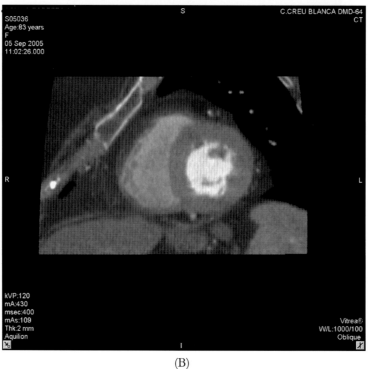

(B)

FIGURE 5.4 Diastolic (A) and systolic (B) frames from a short-axis plane in a normally contracting left ventricle (LV). Observe the homogeneous increase in wall thickness from diastole to systole.

regional systolic dysfunction of ischemic origin[6] (Figure 5.5). Morphological changes in the left ventricle due to chronic coronary artery disease can also be readily depicted, such as the presence of myocardial regions with an abnormally thin wall due to previous infarction[7]

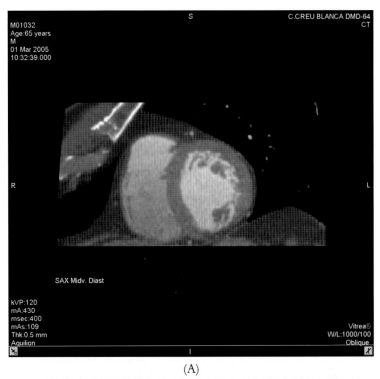

(A)

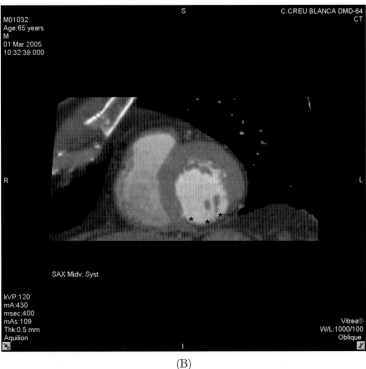

(B)

FIGURE 5.5 Diastolic (A) and systolic (B) frames from a short-axis plane showing a thinned inferior left ventricular wall in diastole without any detectable systolic thickening (asterisks), indicating akinesia due to a previous myocardial infarction.

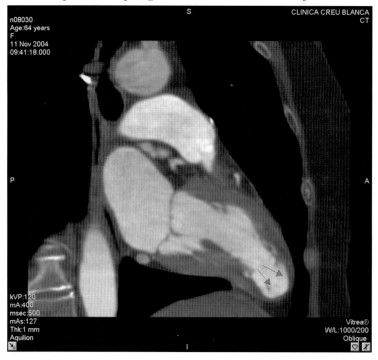

FIGURE 5.6 Systolic frame from a 2-chamber view showing an extremely thin apical region (arrows) protruding in systole, resulting from previous infarction.

(Figure 5.5 and 5.6), left ventricular aneurysm occasionally filled with thrombus (Figure 5.7), or pseudoaneurysm (Figure 5.8).

5.2 Myocardial Tissue Characterization

A wide range of image densities depending on attenuation of X-rays by the different tissues is one of the most useful features of CT studies in general. Densities ranging from the lowest (corresponding to air), to the highest (found on dense bone), can be quantified by the so-called Hounsfield units (HU), a scale that confers levels of density relative to the attenuation imposed by water (HU: 0).

The presence of calcium on any location in the heart is easily identified (Figure 5.9). This constitutes the basis of the detection and quantification of calcium in the coronary arterial wall, which is discussed in a dedicated chapter in this Atlas. However, other subtle signs based on tissue densities can also be found in the heart muscle on a MDCT study. An interesting one is the intriguing finding of areas of myocardial

hypodensity located in regions with a previous myocardial infarction (Figure 5.10). These hypodense areas are observed on noncontrasted scans, such as those performed for the study of coronary calcium, and can be a useful sign for the detection of chronic myocardial necrosis. A proposed explanation for this finding is the process of adipose transformation of the scar after a myocardial necrosis on the long term[8]; as fat gives a low density level on CT scans (negative value of HU), adipose tissues can be distinguished from other soft tissues, which present with slightly higher HU values.

MDCT images after contrast may provide valuable information on myocardial perfusion. In those regions with previous infarction, the presence of a perfusion defect can be detected on the acquisition performed during the arterial phase of the contrast transit[9], the one used for the visualization of the coronary arteries (Figure 5.11). Both animal[10] and clinical[7,11] studies have shown that MDCT is fairly accurate in detecting myocardial infarction by this method, as the mean HU of the infarcted regions is nearly half the value for non-infarcted myocardium, which is around 120 HU. It is important to note that the information on early myocardial perfusion is obtained from the same

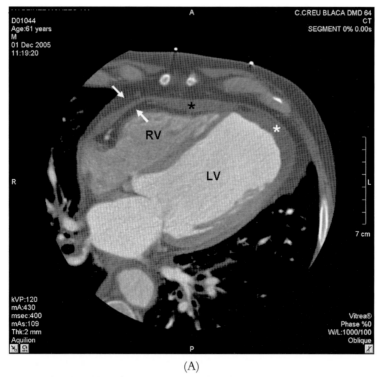

(A)

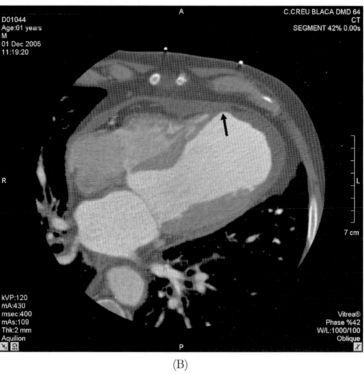

(B)

FIGURE 5.7 Diastolic (A) and systolic (B) frames from a patient with a subacute large anterior myocardial infarction. Note the presence of an aneurysm of the apical portion of the left ventricle (LV) containing a mural thrombus (white asterisk) and, also, a pericardial effusion (black asterisk), clearly distinctive from the epicardial and paracardiac fat (arrows in A) anterior to the right ventricle (RV), and later proved to be of hemorrhagic content. Observe the extensive diskinesia of the apical region and the extremely thinned wall of the most anterior apical segment (arrow in B), probably the site of leakage of intracavitary blood into the pericardial space.

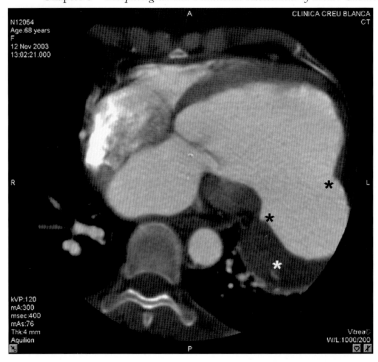

FIGURE 5.8 Axial plane from a patient with a pseudoaneurysm of the lateral left ventricular free wall resulting from a previous infarction. Note the abrupt disruption of the ventricular wall (black asterisks) and a thick laminar thrombus adhered to the inner wall of the pseudoaneurysmal sac (white asterisk).

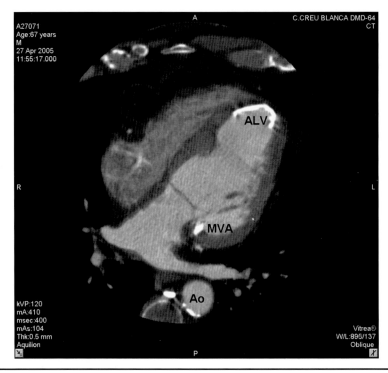

FIGURE 5.9 Axial plane showing three locations of calcium in the cardiovascular structures from different origins: a calcified atherosclerotic aortic plaque (Ao); a calcification of the lateral mitral valve annulus (MVA); and a calcified wall of an apical aneurysm of the left ventricle (ALV).

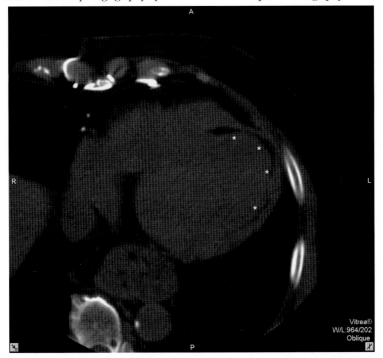

FIGURE 5.10 Axial plane without contrast showing an extensive endocardial area of reduced density at the left ventricular wall (asterisks) in a patient with a previous large anterior myocardial infarction.

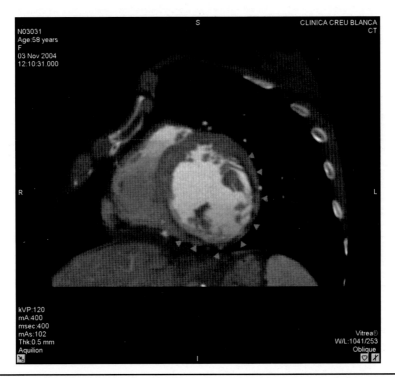

FIGURE 5.11 Short-axis plane with contrast showing reduced attenuation in an extensive subendocardial region of the inferior and lateral left ventricular wall (arrows), indicating a perfusion defect in this area.

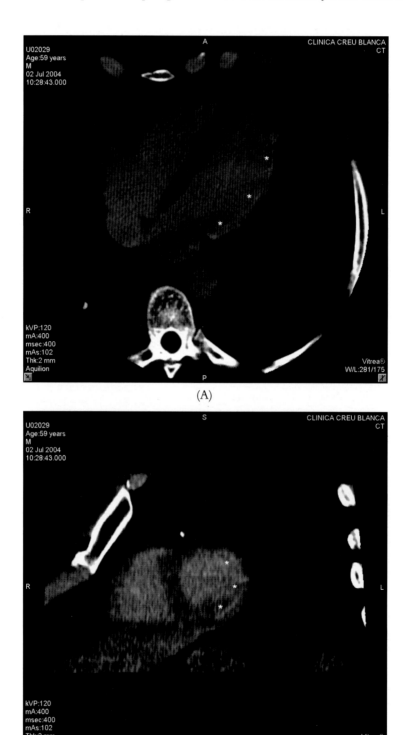

FIGURE 5.12 Longitudinal (A) and short-axis (B) views of a patient with previous anterolateral infarction showing myocardial contrast enhancement (asterisks) in a scan obtained late (5 minutes), after the administration of a conventional iodinated contrast agent.

volume acquired for visualizing the coronary arteries, with no additional radiation.

In addition to this perfusion defect, also, a phenomenon of late contrast enhancement has been described[12,13] (Figure 5.12). Borrowed from CMR studies, the concept of myocardial "late enhancement" refers to the persistence of paramagnetic contrast agents in regions of irreversibly damaged left ventricular myocardium when imaged late (5–15 minutes) after contrast administration. Due to the similar pharmacokinetic properties between iodinated agents and gadolinium compounds, the same mechanism has been proposed for late enhancement: increased volume of distribution in necrotic regions compared with normal myocardium. Studies where both CMR and MDCT have been performed[11] have shown excellent agreement for the estimation of myocardial necrotic mass. Of note, the assessment of myocardial late enhancement by MDCT requires a second acquisition of data minutes after the administration of the iodinated agent, which increases the radiation dose to the patient.

In despite of this, these observations have stimulated interest in the potential value of MDCT in the assessment of myocardial perfusion and viability[14].

Thus, a complete set of information on left ventricular morphology and function, as well as the insight on myocardial perfusion and viability can be obtained on a MDCT examination. As this can be retrieved from the same acquisition that is used for coronary angiography, or adding only a slightly modified strategy, it may allow for an integral study of every patient with coronary artery disease.

References

1. Schuijf, J.D., et al. Noninvasive coronary imaging and assessment of left ventricular function using 16-slice computed tomography. *Am J Cardiol*, 2005, 95, 571–4.

2. Yamamuro, M., et al. Cardiac functional analysis with Multi-Detector Row CT and segmental reconstruction algorithm: comparison with echocardiography, SPECT, and MR imaging. *Radiology*, 2005, 234, 381–90.

3. Schlosser, T., et al. Assessment of left ventricular parameters using 16-MDCT and new software for endocardial and epicardial border delineation. *Am J Röentgenol AJR*, 2005, 184, 765–73.

4. Juergens, K.U., et al. Multi-Detector Row CT of left ventricular function with dedicated analysis software versus MR imaging: initial experience. *Radiology*, 2004, 230, 403–10.

5. Elgeti, T., et al. Comparison of electron beam computed tomography with magnetic resonance imaging in assessment of right ventricular volumes and function. *J Comput Assist Tomogr*, 2004, 28, 679–85.

6. Mahnken, A.H., et al. Acute myocardial infarction: assessment of left ventricular function with 16-detector row spiral CT versus MR imaging—study in pigs. *Radiology*, 2005, 236, 112–7.

7. Nikolaou, K., et al. Assessment of myocardial infarctions using multidetector-row computed tomography. *J Comput Assist Tomogr*, 2004, 28, 286–92.

8. Winer-Muram, H.T., et al. Computed tomography demonstration of lipomatous metaplasia of the left ventricle following myocardial infarction. *J Comput Assist Tomogr*, 2004, 28, 455–8.

9. Hilfiker, P.R., D. Weishaupt, and B. Marincek. Multislice spiral computed tomography of subacute myocardial infarction. *Circulation*, 2001, 104, 1083.

10. Hoffmann, U., et al. Acute myocardial infarction: contrast-enhanced multi-detector row CT in a porcine model. *Radiology*, 2004, 231, 697–701.

11. Mahnken, A.H., et al. Assessment of myocardial viability in reperfused acute myocardial infarction using 16-slice computed tomography in comparison to magnetic resonance imaging. *J Am Coll Cardiol*, 2005, 45, 2042–7.

12. Mochizuki, T., et al. Demostration of acute myocardial infarction by subsecond spiral computed tomography: early defect and delayed enhancement. *Circulation*, 1999, 99, 2058–9.

13. Paul, J.F., et al. Late defect on delayed contrast enhanced multi-detector row CT scans in the prediction of SPECT infarct size after reperfused acute myocardial infarction: initial experience. *Radiology*, 2005, 236, 485–9.

14. Koyama, Y., T. Mochizuki, and J. Higaki. Computed tomographic assessment of myocardial perfusion, viability, and function. *J Magn Reson Imaging*, 2004, 19, 800–15.

Printed in Singapore